YOUR SKIN'S SECRETS

HOW TO RECLAIM YOUR HEALTH AND BANISH CONDITIONS SUCH AS ACNE AND ROSACEA

Marian Rubock

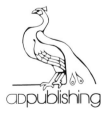

A Self-Published Title
Animal Dreaming Publishing
www.AnimalDreamingPublishing.com

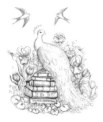

Your Skin's Secrets
Revised Colour Edition

A self-published book produced with the help and support of
ANIMAL DREAMING PUBLISHING
PO Box 5203 East Lismore NSW 2480
AUSTRALIA
Phone +61 2 6622 6147
www.AnimalDreamingPublishing.com
www.facebook.com/AnimalDreamingPublishing

First published in 2016
Revised colour edition published in 2017
Copyright text © Marian Rubock
www.marianrubock.com.au

ISBN 978-0-994524836

Disclaimer
All information in this book is offered for educational purposes only. Please consider and consult professionals in the relevant field to make an educated decision as to whether suggestions in this book are right for you.

I have been fascinated by the human body since I was eight. I remember as a child pulling out our encyclopaedias at home and going straight to the human anatomy section.

This book is the result of many people who have supported me or challenged me to explore what lies beyond and to that I am eternally grateful.

I would like to dedicate this book to those people as well as, my clients, many I have known ten or more years, my family; who said I was headstrong and able to handle any obstacle and my husband who urged me to write my passion down and put it into words.

My mission – to help as many people as I can with skin conditions!

CONTENTS

LIST OF TABLES

LIST OF FIGURES

ABOUT THE AUTHOR

⌒

Marian Rubock is a qualified expert skin care specialist working with skin disorders for the last 15 years. With over thirty-three years of medical experience and having suffered skin disorders herself, Marian has a profound understanding of the skin and how it interacts with your body. She was a columnist on Skin and Beauty issues for *The West Australian* for the last 7 years until October 2013 and is a regular speaker on radio for Curtin FM & a guest at 6PR.

Marian's approach is to take a practical approach to your skin's health by addressing hormonal, nutritional and lifestyle imbalances that affect your health and your skin. By combining advanced medical techniques, including hormonal health, nutrition and natural treatments, she is committed to achieving outstanding results and understanding the causes of skin problems for every client. She understands that we are all different and a 'one size fits all' approach does not apply to the skin.

Marian continues to study the most current and effective natural techniques and innovations in the medical, health and wellbeing sector and leads the way in natural skin health solution development.

MARIAN'S QUALIFICATIONS

Bachelor Degree of Nursing in Applied Science, Deakin University Post Graduate Degree in Occupational Health and Safety, Curtin University Diploma in Operating Room Nursing Management Diploma in Clinical Aromatherapy Diploma in Exercise Physiology and Human Movement Diploma in Massage and Reflexology, Certificate in Homeopathy, Herbal Medicine & Flower Essence, Certificate in Dark-field Microscopy (live blood analysis), Advanced Certificate in Micro-current Therapy.

PROLOGUE

❦

"I have seen everyone for my skin and you are my last hope!" exclaimed Sarah.

Sarah is a young woman in her 30s. She has researched and trialled many skin treatments and has bought nearly every product offered as a cure for her acne, including Acne Medications, antibiotics and over-the-counter treatments, as well as regular peels and exfoliation. Nothing had worked, or it seemed to work for a little while then stopped working, and so here she was sitting in my office, full of hope.

Her acne started after she was put on the contraceptive pill for heavy periods and pain at the age of 14 because she would often miss school for one to two days.

She was a straight-A student at school and went on to university, completing a degree in microbiology. She had good family support, although her dad died of a heart attack unexpectedly when she was 17; she still feels the loss but thinks she copes with it okay. She stated that she expects a lot from herself and others and finds it difficult to be flexible. She admitted to me that she would get anxious and irritated if she could not complete a task and often slept poorly when something was bothering her, waking up tired the next morning..

She had a great job, which she enjoyed, at one of the local hospitals and had just been offered a promotion as team leader in her area. Her long-term boyfriend of two years, had "popped the question" on an overseas holiday and she was looking forward to planning their wedding.

With her skin condition worsening now in her 30s, she was fed up with being female and having sores all over her face. She wasn't looking forward to the wedding pictures, with her face full of acne!

"My diet is pretty good, I think," she said. "I don't eat any fast food, I exercise nearly every day but sometimes I get too tired so I skip, when work is busy. I admit that I forget to drink water on a regular basis and my evening meal is not always healthy food as I come home too tired to cook!"

Sarah's story is a common one. Modern-day living includes changes to how your food is grown, manufactured, processed and packaged. There are conflicting demands on your time; constant stimulation from marketing and our daily use of media; and your body is exposed to petrochemicals from everyday products such as toothpaste, shampoos and personal care products. Your health bears the brunt of all these combined factors. For some of us, including myself, the symptoms of the stresses and imbalances they cause can be seen in your skin.

If this story rings true for you, then maybe you too have an underlying issue that has been missed. Skin conditions such as acne and rosacea are symptoms that your body is out of balance. Come on the journey with me to discover whether your body is in balance and reap the benefits of discovering how to restore your inner health and enjoy beautiful healthy skin!

INTRODUCTION

⁂

Why I wrote this book

I wrote this book for three reasons:

1. I have learned so much about skin conditions in the past 15 years that I wanted to share it with others. I decided to make it my mission to do so.

2. With every new client I see I realise the lack of clear, cohesive information available to teach people how to help themselves and to understand that there is no quick fix for skin health. In reality, nine times out of 10, your skin is the symptom not the cause.

3. I have a deep love and respect for the human body and I am truly amazed at how our body continues on under duress. You see I have suffered acne all my life, but in fact it was my hormones and lack of nutrients that caused the underlying problem. By resolving these issues, I resolved my skin issue.

Let me begin ...

For as long as I can remember I have been fascinated with the workings of our body. This led me to study nursing when I was just shy of 17. It was at this time, in my late teens, that I started to get acne after being diagnosed with a medical condition. For those of you with skin conditions, it will come as no surprise that I was more worried about the acne than I was about my medical condition. I felt ashamed and embarrassed because of my acne. I thought that if I picked at it, it would go away. Whenever anyone spoke to me, I felt as though they were disgusted by my skin and found it hard to look at me.

Thus the journey began to rid myself of this crippling condition. I bought every lotion and potion. I used antibiotics for a while when

I wasn't on them for my medical condition, but still never got any closer to enjoying acne-free skin. Although I was dedicated to achieving the end result, my regular sessions with the beauty therapist never resulted in the healthy, glowing skin I saw in magazines. It was disheartening, but each time I went to have a treatment I lived in hope that this time we would make some progress ...

My obsession with skin grew and I was determined to find the answer to treating acne. I discovered that there is not one magical cure. However, over the past 15 years I have learned some amazing things about your health, your skin and its relationship with the rest of your body.

One overriding element when treating any skin condition is that *your skin is the mirror to your health*. In particular, your hormonal balances, energy and nutrition have an irrefutable impact on your skin's health. Now, in my 50s, my skin is healthy, scar-free, acne-free and better than it's ever been. I look in the mirror with confidence rather than distain and enjoy the feel of my skin, rather than pick at its imperfections!

After treating hundreds of clients over the last 15 years I realised that I wanted them to have all the information that I had. The problem was that I had so much to tell them and so little time to impart it. At this point, one of my clients said to me, "You should write a book, because I won't remember all of this information you are telling me!"

Hence the seed was sown five years ago and today I have completed this writing journey. This book contains valuable information that I know will help you, whether you suffer acne, rosacea, sun damage or if you just want to invest in your skin and health.

This book is designed to help you unlock the jigsaw puzzle of your health and skin. It is no substitute for the support of a qualified practitioner if you need to do further testing and interpret that information.

Marian

How to use this book

This book is divided into three sections to make it easy to use. It is designed to be informative, directive and supportive. I have drawn from my own experiences as an acne sufferer, but also on those of my many clients who have suffered acne, rosacea and other skin complaints. They have been a great source of support and clinical education over the last 15 years.

We all want a natural solution to our skin complaint and to feel confident in ourselves. We are also impatient and by human design want the "quick fix". Unfortunately, there is no such thing and the antibiotics and medications we use, either topically or orally, only mask what is happening deep within our bodies, leaving the problem unaddressed.[1,2,3,5,37,40]

Section One

The first section is an introduction to some of the basic principles of healthy skin.

Section Two

The second section is a resource and discovery area with further explanations about how your body works. There are quick references and assessments, guides, questionnaires and tables to make it easy to understand how various factors affect your skin. Section Two also includes recipes, a food programme as a suggestion for those of you who need to make major overhaul choices to your daily food intake, and diary pages, should you wish to write down what foods or regular habits you have that might be causing stress, intolerances or allergies for your body and skin, also noting when it is at its worst.

Section Three

The third section contains specific information on some of the main skin conditions such as acne, rosacea, and premature ageing and sun damage. In this section there are topical skin care programmes, overhaul checklists for your diet and lifestyle and descriptions of the different types of acne and rosacea. It takes time for your skin to heal and renew itself, so I would suggest that you use the diary in Section Two to help define your day-to-day foods, moods, digestion, energy levels, temperatures and so on, and how it affects your skin. If you monitor your skin for any recurring patterns it will give you a clue to the deeper problem. If you feel as though you are hitting a brick wall, you may choose to find a natural health practitioner to assist you, especially if having completed the questionnaires you decide to do further testing.

I hope you will embrace this book and achieve the results that you aspire to. Enjoy!

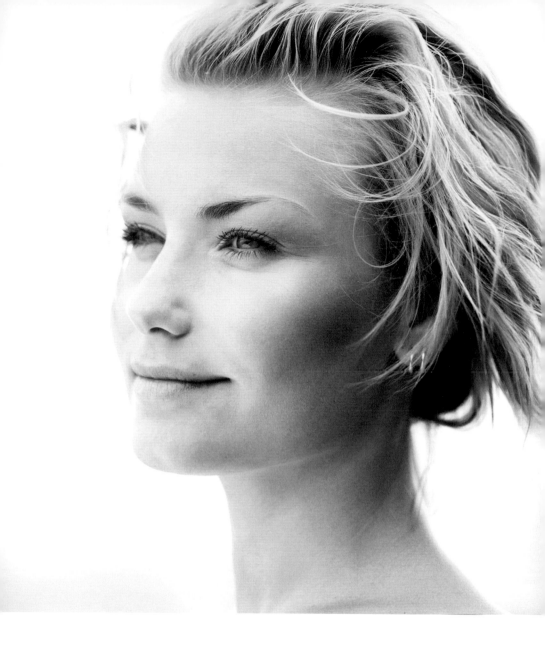

SECTION ONE

YOUR SKIN: WHAT AN AMAZING ORGAN!

☙

Are you aware that your skin, hair and nails are the last organs and structures in your body to get nutrition? This is one of the main reasons, I believe, why we are intuitively drawn towards topical skin care.

From your internal health to your external health, our skin represents a mirror to our chronological ageing as well as our biological ageing. It's our physical body's first line of defence against environmental stresses as well as bacteria, viruses and fungi.

Your skin is vital, not only for your health but also your quality of life. Having healthy skin is no accident or stroke of fate.

Biologically your dermis feeds your epidermis. This means that, like your hair and nails, the top layer of your skin is comprised of dead skin cells and therefore cannot be revitalised — it must get all its nutrients and sustenance from the layer below — your dermis. Using topical vitamins and herbs plays a major role in skin health.[41,43] Your nutritional status also plays an important role in the maintenance of the health of your skin. Macronutrients (carbohydrates, proteins and lipids) and micronutrients (vitamins and nutritionally essential minerals) work together to maintain the barrier of your skin and optimum health to face of everyday challenges. Changes in your nutritional status that alter skin structure and function can also directly affect skin appearance. For example an increase in stress, a bout of gastro causing diarrhoea or training for a marathon/race will require the demand for extra Iodine, magnesium, vitamin C and so on. Unlike many organs, skin nutrition may be enhanced directly through topical applications. Topical application of micronutrients can complement dietary consumption, leading to a stronger, healthier protective barrier for your body.[1,29]

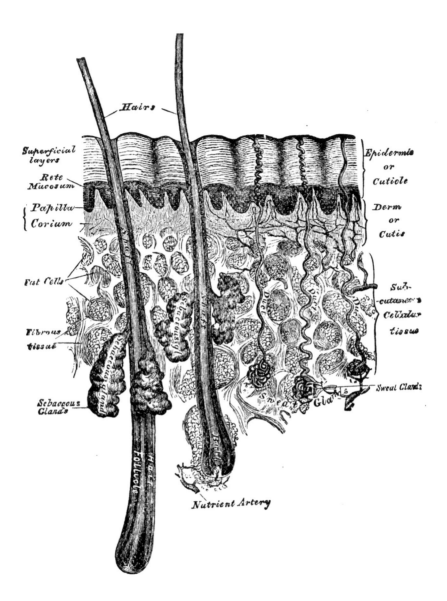

*Figure 1: **Human skin cross section***

Whilst there are a myriad of combinations of vitamins and herbs available, there are certain ones that have a synergy with the skin. When they are presented to the skin in a certain formulation there is maximum absorption and maximum benefit.

Table 1: Vitamin science for your skin

Skin vitamins we like to use	Their skin benefits
Chirally correct skin vitamins	
Vitamin B3	Supports immune function and collagen production.
Biotin, pyridoxine, pantothenic acid	Increases the skin nutrition and blood supply.
Vitamin C (L-ascorbic acid)	Nourishes the skin and helps build collagen and blood supply.
Vitamin A (retinaldehyde — natural is best)	Rebuilds the top layer of skin (the epidermis) and supports the health, hydration and protective functions of the skin. Reverses radiation damage and lines and wrinkles
Vitamin D	Can be used topically where exposure is deficient and is a great support for skin healing. **Clinical note:** *I have also found it very helpful for healing insect bites and rashes.*
Vitamin E	This vitamin resides in the cell walls and helps protect against cellular damage. It also helps rejuvenate vitamin C.
Maximise hydration	
L-hyaluronic acid	Relieves dry skin, accelerates wound healing, rejuvenates ageing skin. Retains moisture of the dermis and epidermis and therefore supports the skin's NMF (natural moisturising factor). May retard premature ageing of the skin, including the photo damage caused by exposure of the skin to ultraviolet radiation.

Skin vitamins we like to use	Their skin benefits
Maximise hydration	
L-hyaluronic acid continued	Facilitates the retention of optimal amounts of water in the matrix of connective tissue in the dermis of the skin (thereby enhancing the elasticity of the skin). Loss of hyaluronic acid depletion (in the dermis) may be one of the underlying causes of wrinkles. Approximately 56% of the body's hyaluronic acid content is present in the skin.
R-lipoic acid, Co enzyme Q10,	All support anti-oxidant damage to the skin's cells.
Amino acids	
L-proline, L-lysine, L-glycine, glutamate, valine, leucine and tryptophan	These are the building blocks for our skin, but due to smoking, stress, coffee, L-histidine, L-methionine, L-cysteine, and ageing, our circulation can be affected. This, in turn, affects our amino acid delivery, thus resulting in poor skin rebuilding.
Fats	
Lipids	Linoleic acid, linolenic acid, cholesterol and phosphatidylcholine.
Fruit exfoliants	
L-mandelic	Derived from almonds, alpha hydroxy acid (AHA) is anti-bacterial, and improves photo-aged skin, acne, abnormal pigmentation, and skin texture.
L-malic	Derived from apples, provides gentle exfoliation, smoothes skin, promotes cellular renewal.

Skin vitamins we like to use	Their skin benefits
Fruit exfoliants	
Actilac™ H-60 (honey extract)	Contains many complex saccharides and oligosaccharides, as well as gluconic acid, which provides moisturising, soothing and conditioning properties.
Peptides	
Matrixyl™ 3000 and SYN®-COLL	Promotes collagen synthesis.
Peptamide™ 6	Firms and tones skin.
Argireline®, Leuphasyl® and SNAP-8	Band together to reduce and prevent wrinkles.
Melanostatine®5	Brightens photo-damaged skin.
Aldenine®	Protects against further harmful UV damage.
Anti-inflammatory, protective	
Zinc oxide	Broad-spectrum protection from UVA and UVB exposure, which also promotes healing, soothes and calms the skin.
Thiotaine®	Natural antioxidant and amino acid, prevents damage caused by UV radiation, recycles vitamin C, assures efficient energy production, inhibits tyrosinase.
Porphyra umbilicalis (red algae) extract	Organism that lives in shallow water where it is exposed to extreme UV radiation, produces the most powerful UV-absorbing substances in nature, and the extract itself absorbs both UVA and UVB light.
Olea europaea (olive) fruit oil*	Rich in vitamin E and antioxidants that replace skin moisture and elasticity, it is anti-inflammatory and anti-bacterial.

Skin vitamins we like to use	Their skin benefits
Miscellaneous Nutrients	
Pomegranate, rosehip, Kakadu plum, blackcurrant and pumpkin oils	Enriched with vitamins A, B and C, essential for the formation of proline, an amino acid required to make collagen.

As you can see, there are a great number of vitamins that will benefit your skin as well as herbs, more of which will be discussed in Section Three.

Clinical note:

"In my early years of practising I thought that all skin vitamins were equal. When I decided to research and invest in my own skin care range I understood the power of the term "chirally correct". When products are chirally correct, they are produced to the right formulation for absorption by the skin and provide maximum benefit. This means that they reach the dermis where it can improve the health of your skin.

One of my clients captures the benefits of my products being chirally correct and the impact these have had on her skin's health, with the following words:

I have had dry skin to the point of being painful. I know it is because I did too much sun tanning as a teenager, but we didn't know how harmful it was then. Feel my skin; it feels moist for the first time and I am so pleased that finally I have found some products that work!"

Based on the knowledge that healthy skin is not achieved by accident, if you have a skin disorder you will appreciate how important it is to understand the basic principles that result in healthy skin. When your body is undernourished, overstressed and dehydrated through day-to-day life your skin, whilst it is the largest organ of your body, gets its nutrients last! Therefore, ensuring that your skin gets fed every day, so to speak, is vital if you want to have healthy skin during your 20s, 30s, 40s and beyond. This will also reduce the risk of premature ageing and various skin conditions, including sun damage and abnormalities such as solar keratosis. The quality and type of skin care you choose, as well as your personal care products and make-up, on a day-to-day basis, will have an accumulative effect, either towards your skin's ageing in future years or its health.

Five basic principles of healthy skin

The **five** basic principles of healthy skin are:

1. The **quality of the skin care** you use, its formulation and your dedication to your regime. Your skin care needs to support and feed your dermis (second layer of skin) and the epidermis (top layer).

2. The **quality of the food you eat** and its nutrient base as well as your body's ability to absorb those nutrients. Food can be an allergen in your body and cause inflammation at a very low level. Often this is when your skin will flare up periodically, with conditions such as acne and rosacea. If you are low on certain nutrients and your diet has been high in processed sugars, your body will be nutritionally stressed and this will affect the long-term functionality of your body and metabolism. In particular, stress affects your adrenal glands, reproductive hormones and thyroid — your body's engine driver.

3. The **quality, amount and depth of sleep** you get each night is important as your body completes its housework, so to speak.[1,4,31,34] Sleep rebalances your hormonal glands, optimises your digestive system, and realigns your body to optimise function for the next day so you can be at your best. Contrary to popular belief, you cannot catch up on sleep. If you are having short sleeps, don't be fooled into thinking you will catch up later. If you are consistently waking up tired, then try changing your habits before bed; avoid alcohol, caffeine and energy drinks; reduce your exposure to bright lights such as TVs and computers, and reduce the heating thermostat in your bedroom.[4,22,32,33] Restful sleep is beauty sleep. All the top models and actors know this, which is why they are very disciplined in their sleep patterns.

I once read that Jennifer Anniston goes to bed at 9.30 pm every night and gets up at about 5 am to do her exercise regime before she starts the day!

4. Whilst the **accumulative effect of your lifestyle choices** is important, so too are the conversations you have with yourself. When you were in your mother's womb, the same cells, which are now your skin cells, also transformed into nerve cells[45]. This creates a powerful connection between your nervous system, and skin. To give you an example of this connection, imagine how your skin responds when you are embarrassed: your skin will flush.

5. The consistent **balance within your blood sugar/digestive hormones, sex hormones, stress and metabolic hormones,** all of which play a role in the health of your skin and how it responds externally as well as its long-term health.

You can read more about this in Section Two.

What quality skin care should provide

To improve, renew and reverse skin damage, your skin needs skin care that will do the following:

1. **Cleanse without stripping the skin** — this is to maintain a healthy pH, remove debris and make-up for healthy skin, and to support skin immunity.

2. **Remodel** — this removes scarring, resurfaces the epidermis by supplying nutrients to the dermis, reduces inflammation, supports epidermal moisture, and re-establishes free fatty acids, cholesterol and ceramides.

3. **Feed and nourish** — this supports the day-to-day requirements of your skin and busy lifestyle through chirally correct natural nutrition that sinks deep into the dermis.

4. **Moisturise** — this supports a healthy epidermis to reduce dermal ageing, thinning and dehydration. In particular, after the age of 40 there is a sharp decline in skin lipids, thus increasing your susceptibility to dry skin conditions. The decreases in lipids may also be due to a low functioning thyroid.

5. **Protect** — this reduces sun damage, ageing from radiation trauma and prevention of solar keratosis and sun-induced skin disorders.[43]

With so many products on the market, I am sure you feel inundated and find it hard to know which one to choose. I know from my own experience that every time I bought something new, not only could I not wait to try it, but the hope that it would fix my acne was foremost in my mind.

I have found through my own and my clients' experience that not all skin products are equal. It may surprise you, tongue in cheek, that often the cost of the jar is more expensive than the actual combination of ingredients inside it!

With this in mind, I wanted to find a skin product that did what it promised to do and my list of requirements was long. A skin product should be:

- a pure product and not full of fillers
- not tested on animals
- naturally derived
- results-driven.

It must not contain:

- no proven harsh skin irritant ingredients and petrochemicals
- no parabens
- no xenoestrogens, which cause hormone disruption and cause more skin problems!
- no nasties.

Most importantly, it must consist of a low molecular weight in order to get into the deeper layers of skin to *feed the dermis!*

There is more on skin care in Section Three.

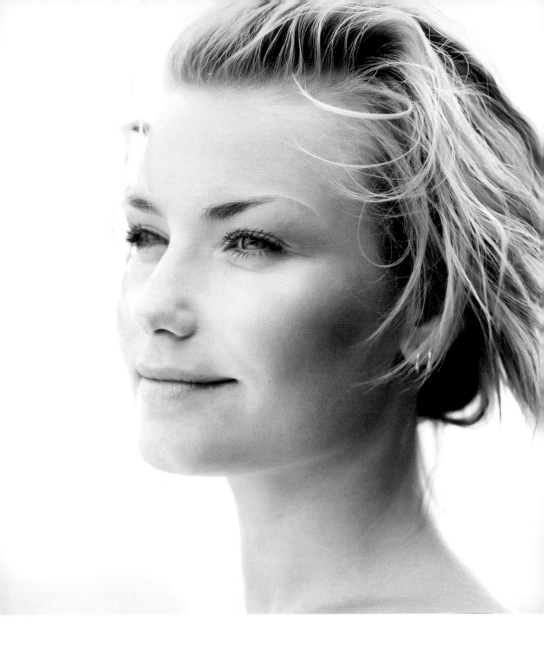

SECTION TWO

This section is designed to be a resource to help you understand a little more about your skin and how it works in conjunction with the rest of your body. You may scan through it and go to the sections you are concerned about to find out what might be the cause of your skin problem. Alternatively, do the questionnaires to learn more, and use the diary section to record your diet, what you are eating and your lifestyle habits, such as stress, moods and activities such as intense exercise. Note how much you are ingesting in the way of stimulants such as coffee, tea, energy drinks and alcohol, and your sleep patterns and/or lack of sleep. It is important as these all factor into what is happening in your body.

I have included a meal plan with recipes to help you through the difficult initial changes as they are often when you are least likely to succeed due to feeling overwhelmed and confused.

In the last 30-plus years, I have learned that often the resistant skin problems are a symptom rather than a condition on their own. So, if you have changed your diet, and are applying quality, natural skin care, with no harmful ingredients, and having removed some of the stimulants that affect your skin such as dairy, sugar and stress, then we need to look deeper. The next section is designed as a resource to help you discover and define what your body may be missing to help you add those ingredients. If you are going to go it alone to start with, it is important that you keep a diary so you can see patterns as they will give you vital clues for what to do next.

It's also important that you give your body time to heal if you are implementing something new. Your skin is a living organ, not a machine, and it takes time for the body to heal and make new changes.

If you are aged 0–25 years, each renewal cycle of your skin is approximately 30 days.

If you are aged 25–40, your renewal cycle is approximately 45 days and if you are over 40, the renewal cycle is approximately 60 days.

So, let's get started.

YOUR SKIN AND YOUR HORMONAL HEALTH: THE COMPLEX CONNECTION

Your skin is an amazing organ, weighing in at about 7 kg for the average adult. It is the largest organ of the body and responsible for many activities to ensure mental and physical health.[41] It is your first line of defence against invading bacteria and viruses as well as environment stresses such as wind, rain, sun and so on. It functions also as an excretory organ, removing toxins from our body by our sebaceous and sweat glands as I am sure you have noticed when you exercise.

The other systems of your body that are involved in your first line of defence are your mouth and digestive system, which is why I will talk about the benefits of "oil pulling"[44] on page 76 and your nose and respiratory tract.

When it comes to your skin's health, you may already have some understanding, especially if you are female, that your hormones play an important role in your skin's health.[3,34,40]

Without getting too technical, let me explain: in your skin there are many structures. Two components that you may have heard about that are involved in skin conditions such as acne and rosacea are your sebaceous glands and your skin's natural moisturising factor, or NMF for short.

We will focus on these two components for now as we discuss how your stress levels affect these structures and mirror the effects of stress on your skin.

Research[45] has shown that an increase in stress hormones made by your adrenal glands, in response to stress, inhibits lipid production in your skin, therefore affecting not only the skin's resilience as a barrier but also its hydration. This means that your skins dermis is then under further stress as your epidermis demands more support.

Good hydration is imperative for healthy skin as the skin's cells need to fold, move and maintain adherence as they move with your body. A continual change or decrease in hydration can lead to trauma and injury to the skin, leaving your skin, and your health, in a vulnerable state.

Your sebaceous glands, which are located in your dermis, are hormonally driven glands that respond to your stress, and reproductive and metabolic hormones. Sebaceous glands are holocrine glands found over the entire surface of the body except the palms, soles and dorsum of the feet. They are largest and most concentrated in the face and scalp where they are the sites of acne when they are working ineffectively. The normal function of sebaceous glands is to produce and secrete sebum, a group of complex oils including triglycerides and fatty acid breakdown products, wax esters, squalene, cholesterol esters and cholesterol. Sebum lubricates the skin to protect against friction and makes it more impervious to moisture, therefore enhancing and supporting your skin's normal hydration.

Furthermore, the sebaceous gland transports antioxidants in and on the skin and exhibits a natural, light, protective activity. It possesses an innate antibacterial activity and has a pro- and anti-inflammatory function. It can regulate the activity of xenobiotics and is actively involved in the wound healing process of your skin. So you can see how important it is to have healthy functioning sebaceous glands.

In addition, there are other hormonal glands in your body that have an effect on your skin and overall health; collectively these are called your Endocrine system.

- **adrenal glands** — responsible for fight and flight as well as the production of over 50 other hormones and enzymes affecting every cell in your body
- **thyroid gland** — your body's engine and regulator with receptors that affect the skin, hair, reproduction, adrenal glands and in fact every cell in your body
- **reproductive glands** — with receptors in your adrenal glands, thyroid gland, skin, brain and so on
- **hypothalamus** and **anterior** and **posterior pituitary,** which are in your brain and are all part of your endocrine system.

ENDOCRINE SYSTEM

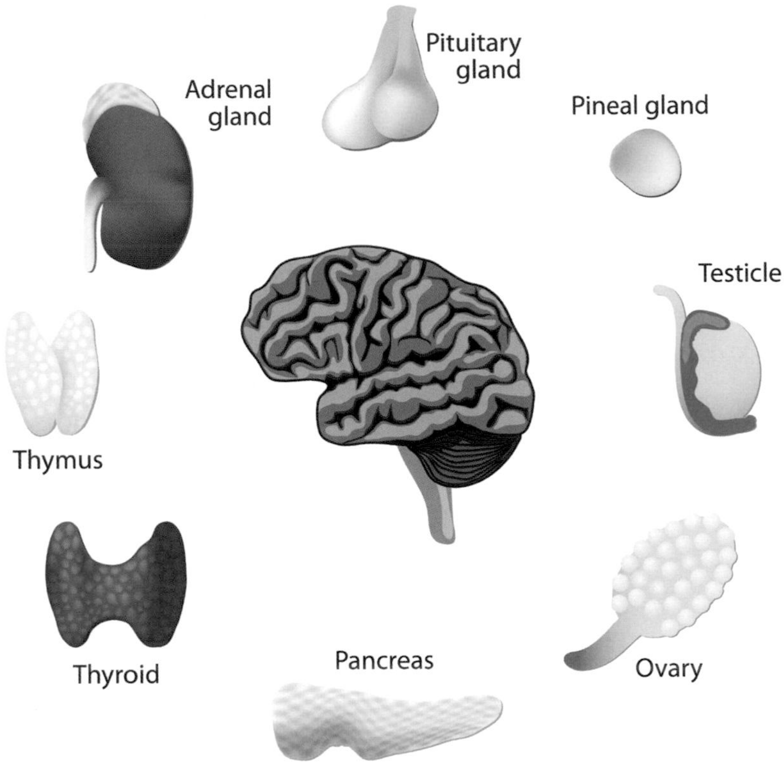

Pituitary
gland

Adrenal
gland

Pineal gland

Testicle

Thymus

Thyroid

Pancreas

Ovary

Figure 2: The glands that make up your endocrine system

Are all these hormonal glands and their harmonious interaction vital to healthy functioning skin and a healthy body? The answer is a resounding YES!

If you have already tried diet-based changes and your skin problems still exist, I would suggest that you reassess your diet. There are some modifications in my recommendations that you may not have implemented as yet and, if you are female, monitor your menstrual cycle, to see when in your cycle you see skin changes or worsening.

If you are taking the contraceptive pill and getting skin changes/breakouts/flushing, then I would suggest you also take your basal metabolic temperature. *(See the information on your thyroid gland on page 38 and basal metabolic temperature chart on page 47.)*

Even though the contraceptive pill has been designed for skin breakouts, some females are sensitive to this medication and rather than improve your skin health the increase in oestrogen has the ability to affect the oestrogen receptors in the thyroid, ovaries and adrenal glands, causing an imbalance and either no change in acne or a worsening.[3,40] If your oestrogen becomes elevated and out of balance with your other hormones it may supress your thyroid function and therefore your skin's health and renewal cycle, resulting in acne, flushing and other skin complaints such as rashes and dry skin patches in both males and females. These affects may be amplified if your liver is unable to cope with your body's detoxification needs – more about that in the digestive section.

Some other factors that affect your skin and endocrine system are:

- pesticides
- halogens, namely ***fluorine, chlorine and bromine*** (these chemicals compete with iodine at the receptor sites for your thyroid. Bromide affects healthy oestrogen metabolism and has been linked to Polycystic ovary disease. You can also find some of these chemicals in your toothpaste, mouthwash and drinking water. Opt for fluoride-free toothpaste and mouthwashes and filter your water)
- mercury
- excessive alcohol
- cigarette smoking
- low adrenal function
- regular use of opiates such as codeine
- medications such as beta blockers, phenytoin, antidepressants
- low nutritional status such as vitamin D, zinc, iodine and amino acids — often more significant with a vegetarian diet.

YOUR ADRENAL HEALTH

ॐ

Your stress response is a normal and necessary response for your survival. However, in our modern way of living we tend to use our stress response on a day-to-day basis and are exhausting our body using our expensive fight and flight response for day-to-day activities and maintaining body balance, rather than survival.

Before the technological and industrial boom we were, as a race, much more active and when your body responded to stress and released adrenal and cortisol hormones, these were burned up through activity and exercise in the course of your day. Now, because of the increase in your automated and more sedentary lifestyle, the adrenal and cortisol hormones that are released at stressful events you may be experiencing— which can be mental, emotional or physical, for example a negative comment sent to you by text — are not as easily eliminated from your body, especially if you are experiencing many of these. With this becoming a constant way of life it has the potential to be extremely damaging to your cells in all areas of your body. *(See the symptoms of stress on page 37.)*

High or low cortisol levels are associated with skin conditions such as acne, rosacea[45], weight gain, hypothyroidism and hair loss. With an imbalance in cortisol comes an imbalance in your sex/reproductive and metabolic hormones such as progesterone, testosterone, oestrogen and thyroxin.[1-3,12,34,42] This causes a subtle chaos within your digestive system and general health as your body struggles to maintain balance.

Acne or flushing that is worse within days 10–16 of your menstrual cycle will often suggest that your progesterone is low, implying that you are oestrogen-dominant and there is not enough progesterone to balance the two hormones or your thyroid is being suppressed. By completing a diary, it is beneficial to define where the problem lies. If your symptoms are worse towards the end of your cycle and your skin feels rough and dry with slow or poor healing, your acne/skin condition may then be related to low testosterone, which for one balances the oestrogen receptors in your thyroid gland, indicating that your thyroid may be working below par. *(See the thyroid checklist on page 40, 41)*

Keeping a basal metabolic temperature chart (taking your temperature first thing in the morning before getting out of bed) and analysing it over a month will help you see if there is a problem with your thyroid and metabolic health. *(See the information regarding thyroid health on page 38 to learn more.)*

So, what are the symptoms of stress and what would indicate that you should get further testing?

The effects of stress are very individual and do vary from one person to another, but generally fall into four categories: behavioural; cognitive, related to thinking, rationalising and reflecting; emotional; and physical.[3]

Behavioural symptoms:

- ☐ Compulsive eating
- ☐ Critical attitude
- ☐ Difficulty in completing tasks
- ☐ Disrupted sleep
- ☐ Grinding teeth while asleep
- ☐ Increased alcohol consumption
- ☐ Neglecting responsibilities
- ☐ Smoking or drug use
- ☐ Short temper

Cognitive symptoms:

- ☐ Anxious or racing thoughts
- ☐ Constant worry and/or ruminating
- ☐ Forgetfulness
- ☐ Inability to make decisions
- ☐ Negativity
- ☐ Poor judgement
- ☐ Poor mental clarity or thinking clearly

Emotional symptoms:

- ☐ Anger — You feel angry but you are not sure why
- ☐ Anxiety
- ☐ Apathy or boredom
- ☐ Depression
- ☐ Easily upset
- ☐ Feeling easily overwhelmed or powerless
- ☐ Loneliness
- ☐ Moodiness

Physical symptoms:

- ☐ Aches and pains
- ☐ Bowel movement irregularities or diagnosed with irritable bowel syndrome
- ☐ Chest pain
- ☐ Decreased interest in sex
- ☐ Dizziness
- ☐ Fatigue
- ☐ Headaches
- ☐ Indigestion
- ☐ Nausea
- ☐ Rapid heart rate
- ☐ Ringing in the ears, also known as tinnitus
- ☐ Weight gain

If you have ticked several of these symptoms, stress may be part of your skin problem and it would be worthwhile considering a stress saliva test to check the health of your adrenal glands. If you would like to check your adrenal hormonal health, the gold standard is a collection of four samples of saliva over a 12-hour period to be sent to a functional medicine laboratory for analysis.

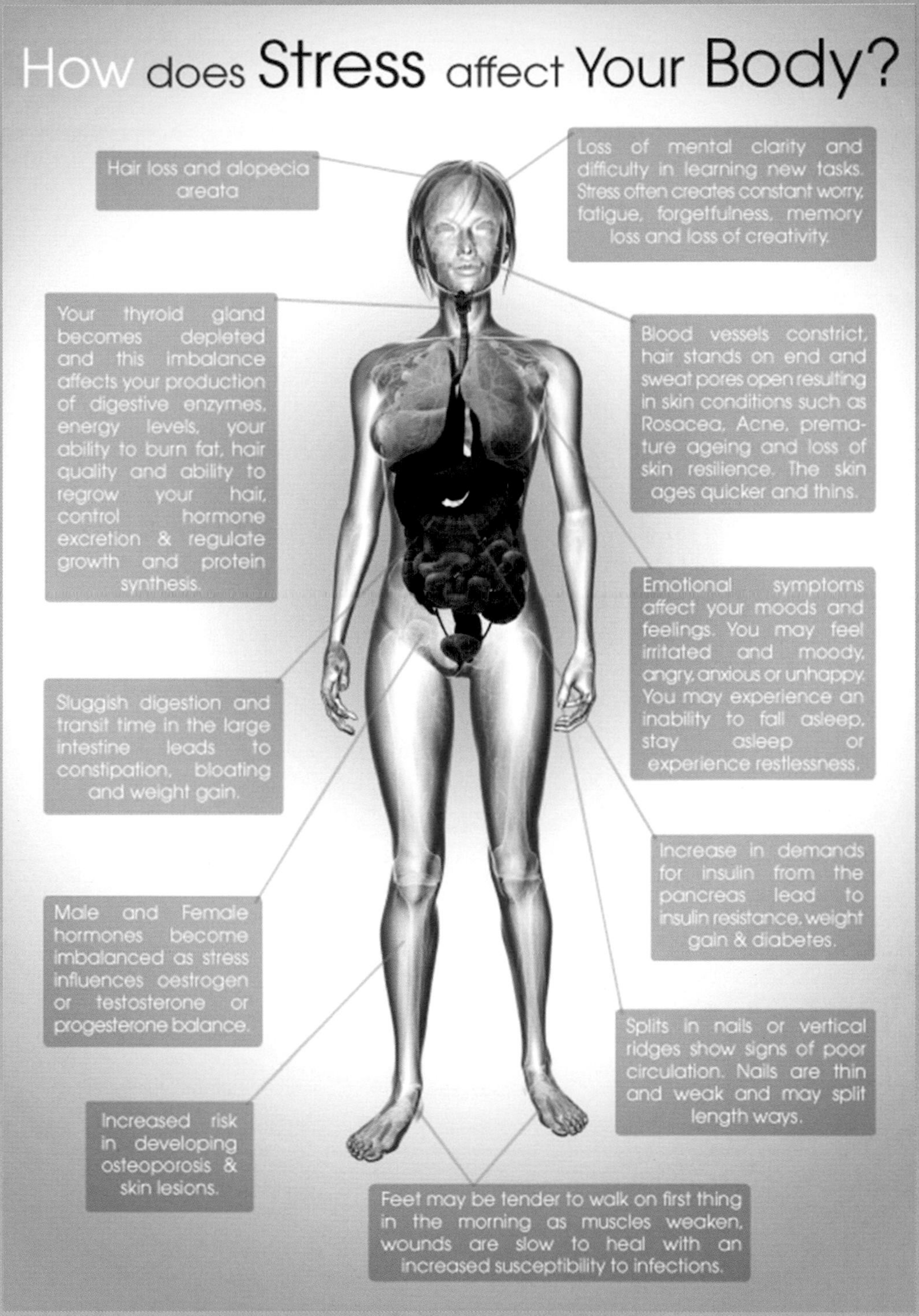

How does Stress affect Your Body?

Hair loss and alopecia areata

Loss of mental clarity and difficulty in learning new tasks. Stress often creates constant worry, fatigue, forgetfulness, memory loss and loss of creativity.

Your thyroid gland becomes depleted and this imbalance affects your production of digestive enzymes, energy levels, your ability to burn fat, hair quality and ability to regrow your hair, control hormone excretion & regulate growth and protein synthesis.

Blood vessels constrict, hair stands on end and sweat pores open resulting in skin conditions such as Rosacea, Acne, premature ageing and loss of skin resilience. The skin ages quicker and thins.

Emotional symptoms affect your moods and feelings. You may feel irritated and moody, angry, anxious or unhappy. You may experience an inability to fall asleep, stay asleep or experience restlessness.

Sluggish digestion and transit time in the large intestine leads to constipation, bloating and weight gain.

Increase in demands for insulin from the pancreas lead to insulin resistance, weight gain & diabetes.

Male and Female hormones become imbalanced as stress influences oestrogen or testosterone or progesterone balance.

Splits in nails or vertical ridges show signs of poor circulation. Nails are thin and weak and may split length ways.

Increased risk in developing osteoporosis & skin lesions.

Feet may be tender to walk on first thing in the morning as muscles weaken, wounds are slow to heal with an increased susceptibility to infections.

Figure 3: How stress affects your body

YOUR THYROID HEALTH

❧

To check your thyroid gland and its health, you can get a blood test, but make sure you request T4, T3 and Reverse T3 so you can identify the functioning of your thyroid. The test will ascertain not just if it is getting all the right signals from the brain, but, more importantly, how efficiently it is working when it receives those signals.

Another moderately accurate way you can check your thyroid health is by taking and recording your basal metabolic temperature first thing in the morning before you get out of bed. A normal thyroid should sit around 36.5° Celsius or 97.7° Fahrenheit when taken under the armpit daily. If you are a menstruating female, it is normal for your temperature to rise slightly around days 11–16 of your 28-day cycle.

The main nutrient that allows your thyroid to work efficiently is iodine, being closely supported by zinc and vitamin D. The problem for your thyroid is that iodine is disappearing from our food supply, combined with exposure to the family of halogens (bromine, fluorine, chlorine and perchlorate), which has dramatically increased.[2,12,14,15] These halogens are absorbed into our body through your food, water, medications and the environment, and they selectively occupy your iodine receptors, further deepening your iodine deficit and affecting your health, weight management, mental health and skin.[12]

Fluoridation of water is a major contributor to iodine deficiency, besides being very damaging to your health in many other ways.

Additional factors contributing to falling iodine levels are:[50,51]

- diets low in fish, shellfish and seaweed (eating farmed fish does not increase iodine levels)
- vegan and vegetarian diets

- decreased use of iodised salt and salt in general
- less use of iodide in the food and agricultural industry
- use of radioactive iodine in many medical procedures, which competes with natural iodine.

So, if you find your temperature is low over the next month of assessment, what should you do?

The chances are that your iodine is low and possibly your thyroid is working below optimum as a result, as discussed above, there may be a variety of factors causing this; however, one way to start to reverse the damage and support a healthy metabolism and healthy skin is to replace the iodine.

Firstly, let's confirm that you are iodine-deficient. The best way to evaluate your iodine intake is a test that measures how much iodine you are excreting in your urine.

The general protocol requires you to take a dose of iodine, collect your urine for 24 hours, and then send the sample off to a laboratory where they calculate your iodine level based on how much iodine you are spilling into your urine. It is called the iodine challenge test and is the best way to objectify if you are deficient.

In the meantime while you are waiting for results you can improve your dietary sources by including seaweed, garlic, asparagus or kelp on a daily basis. However, Dr David Brownstein[14] discusses that often to start with dietary sources may not be enough and a supplement of 10 mg or more may be needed to create a healthy thyroid function. Other sources of iodine are iodised salt, cod, Irish moss, lima beans, mushrooms, oysters and sunflower seeds.

Factors that increase[5] the need for **more** iodine in your diet are: excessive diarrhoea, excessive carbohydrate intake such as your processed foods, excessive weight gain and/or difficulty in losing weight, pregnancy, presence of a goitre, eating a excessive amounts of goitrogen-rich foods such as cabbage, turnips, Brussels sprouts, broccoli, cauliflower, soy and cassava.

David Brownstein[14] has written several books on thyroid and iodine, which are a valuable resource for those of you who want more information.

If you are wondering whether you have a thyroid dysfunction, consider the following symptoms to see if they are relevant to you. If you are experiencing several of these, together with your basal metabolic temperature being low, I would suggest starting some iodine and/or increasing iodine-rich foods into your diet, continuing to monitor your temperature and consider an iodine challenge test. If you are improving the health of your thyroid, your basal metabolic temperature (under the arm) will increase, (if low to start with), and normalise to 36.5° Celsius or 97.7° Fahrenheit. Be patient with yourself as it may take 6–12 months. Keeping a journal is the best way to see changes and improvement as well as in your skin.

Symptoms of an unhealthy thyroid are:

- Acne
- Allergies
- Anaemia
- Anxiety
- Bladder and kidney Infections
- Bone loss
- Brittle nails
- Carpal tunnel syndrome
- Cold hands and cold feet
- Cold Intolerance
- Constipation
- Depressed reflexes
- Depression
- Difficulty in concentrating
- Dizziness
- Downturned mouth
- Droopy eyelids
- Dry, course or thinning hair
- Dry, itchy ear canals
- Dull facial expression
- Easy bruising
- Eating disorder
- Erectile dysfunction

- Excess ear wax
- Fatigue
- Fluid retention
- Goitre (enlarged thyroid)
- Headaches
- Hoarse, husky voice
- Increase in appetite
- High cholesterol
- Insomnia
- Irritability
- Longer, heavier, or more frequent periods
- Loss of hair on arms, legs or underarms
- Low blood pressure
- Low blood sugar
- Low sex drive
- Memory loss
- Muscle and joint pain
- Muscle weakness
- Night-time incontinence
- Numbness and tingling of the extremities
- Poor circulation
- Poor night vision
- Puffy face
- Reduced heart rate
- Rough, dry skin
- Sleep apnoea
- Slow speech
- Swollen legs, feet, hands or abdomen
- Tennis elbow
- Thinning or loss of eye lashes
- Tinnitus
- Vitamin B12 deficiency
- Weight gain
- Yellow skin

Also, Dr Hyman[15] has made some good recommendations if you have a sluggish thyroid:

- Identify and treat the underlying causes (for example, iodine deficiency, hormone imbalance, environmental toxicity, inflammation). Remember that aluminium affects the health of your thyroid, so make sure you throw out those underarm sprays containing aluminium and check all your other personal care products.
- Adjust your diet and understand the role of nutrition (iodine, as well as tyrosine, selenium, vitamins A, D and B complex, zinc, and omega-3 fats), food allergies, gluten intolerance, and foods that contain goitrogens, such as soy, which interfere with the utilisation of iodine.
- Get plenty of exercise.
- Get eight to nine hours of sleep a night.
- Reduce your stress.
- Enjoy saunas and hot soaks for detoxification — with reduced chloride exposure.
- Use supplements, where necessary for nutritional support.
- Eliminate or reduce your exposure to halides that compete with iodine and affect your thyroid's health. Halides such as Bromide; found in bread and other pastries and pastas; Fluoride found in toothpaste, drinking water, etc; and chloride found in spas swimming pools and bleaches.

Laura Power[15] offers these suggestions for increasing secretion of fluorine and bromine:

- Consume high-dose iodine.
- Consume high-dose vitamin C.
- Use unrefined sea salt.
- Soak in Epsom salts baths.
- Sweat in a far-infrared sauna.

Remember: If your temperature is low and you start increasing foods containing iodine, make sure you continue to take and chart your temperature so you can see if the actions you are taking are making a difference. Give your body time to heal as it may take 6–12 months. If you are having difficulty or are unsure, it is best to find a natural therapist to assist you and consider testing.

There are various factors to consider that, apart from being nutritionally low in iodine, will also contribute to low thyroid levels:

- Ageing
- Alcohol abuse
- Dioxins
- Elevated lipoic acid
- Excess copper (such as copper pipes)
- Heavy metal toxicity
- High fluoride levels
- Insufficient DHEA
- Medications including beta blockers, birth control pills, chemotherapy, oestrogen, lithium, phenytoin and theophylline
- PCBs
- Pesticides
- Phthalates
- Radiation
- Stress
- Surgical removal of thyroid

Are you lacking iodine?

Iodine-deficient soil: Australia, India and several African and European countries have geographical areas of severe iodine deficiency[50]. They are usually located long distances from the sea. Deficiency may also be caused by erosion, desertification, flooding and soil overuse.[47,48]

Food sourced from inland areas with no access to sea-sourced foods: This particularly applies to poor people who cannot afford fish or seaweed in their diets.

Eating a modern diet, high in processed foods: Iodine was added to commercial baking as a dough conditioner in the 1960's in an effort to increase iodine levels that were noted to have declined by 50% over the last 30 years[14] however some researchers felt that this of iodine may cause problems with thyroid function and so 20 years later Bromide is used to replace iodine. Unfortunately we know that halides compete with one another and as a result the substitute of bromide for iodine in the bakery process has become another factor in iodine depletion.

Health diets: Many so-called healthy diets are very low in iodine. If you are a vegetarian you are at high risk. Sea salt contains virtually no iodine. If you (sensibly) avoid processed salt and other processed foods, it is essential to eat plenty of kelp/kombu, or to supplement iodine.

Goitrogens: Goitrogens are substances/foods that prevent the uptake of iodine by the thyroid gland and in the rest of the body. Our exposure to goitrogens is much higher than 50 or more years ago. Their primary effect is suppressed thyroid function. Grasses are some of the most potent goitrogens, such as millet (grass seed) and bamboo shoots. The two main food categories of goitrogens are cruciferous vegetables and soybeans. Crucifers include broccoli, cabbage, cauliflower, brussels sprouts, mustard, rutabagas, kohlrabi and turnips. Soy foods include soy milk, tofu, tempeh and TVP. Other goitrogenic foods include peach, strawberry, peanut and spinach. Goitrogens are also prevalent as halogens in the water supply and environment. Fluorides are added to the water supply, toothpaste and some medications in some countries, in the mistaken belief that they strengthen teeth. Research shows that fluorides lead to behavioural disorders, hypothyroidism, hip fractures, bone cancer and kidney damage. Bromine is used as a fire retardant, in carpets and clothing, in the preparation of white baking flour, as an antibacterial agent, as a fumigant and pesticide, in the manufacture of some carbonated drinks, and in some pharmaceuticals. Chlorine is added to drinking water as a disinfectant and used to bleach our wheat flour white, and has been linked to heart disease and cancer.

Remember: the following situations may require you to consume more than the regular daily intake (RDI) of iodine:

- increased stress
- increased consumption of refined carbohydrates
- regular episodes of diarrhoea (more than three per week) as in irritable bowel, Chrohn's disease and diverticulitis
- increased exercise intensity
- pregnancy.

Complete the questionnaire below and *if you score higher than eight* you should consider having your iodine levels checked by a health care professional. In Australia, the gold standard for iodine level testing is a 24 hour urine collection. Check in your own country to see if this is available for you.

Rate your symptoms from 0 to 3.

None = 0   Mild = 2   Moderate = 2   Severe = 3

____ Tired and sluggish

____ Dry hair and skin

____ Increase in need for sleep

____ Weak muscles

____ Constantly feeling cold (fingers)

____ Frequent muscle cramps

____ Poor memory

____ Depressed

____ Slow thinking

____ Slow speech

____ Puffy face or eyes

____ Hoarser or deeper voice, especially in the morning

____ Difficulty with maths

____ Muscle or joint pain

____ Constipation

____ Coarser hair or hair loss

____ Low sex drive or impotence

____ Puffy hands or feet

____ Unsteady gait

____ Gain weight easily

____ Thinning of the outer eyebrow

____ Enlarged tongue

____ Goitre bulge or band around the neck

____ Do you use salt with iodine Yes = 0 or No = 1

For women only to complete the next three questions

____ Is your menses/period more irregular >28 days?

____ Do you have heavy bleeding?

____ Do you have fibrocystic breasts/breast lumps/ovarian cysts?

Total score _____

Number of days you eat shellfish/seafood _____

Your basal metabolic temperature chart

A quick check for your thyroid gland and ongoing monitoring

Remember you must take your temperature first thing in the morning before you get out of bed as once you start moving around the temperature result will be inaccurate.

Preferably use a digital thermometer and place it under your arm. Wait until it sounds the alarm then document your temperature on the chart. For a healthy thyroid, you will need to sit around 36.5° Celsius or 97.7° Fahrenheit. It is best to monitor your temperature (males and females) for at least one month, as there are peaks that occur at certain times within this four-week period. If you are constantly below 36.5° Celsius or 97.7° Fahrenheit, start with changing your diet, removing the toxic load from your body, removing halogens such as fluoride, chloride and any possible xenoestrogens. Consider another contraceptive programme than the contraceptive pill and stabilise your insulin levels with your diet as well as remove processed foods and foods high in processed simple sugars such as chocolates, lollies, energy drinks, fruit juices. If you are still floundering, seek the help of a trained natural health practitioner to help you check and restore your thyroid health.

Table 2: Basal metabolic temperature chart

Temperature in degrees Celsius	Date	1	2	3	4	5	6	7	8	9	10	11	12	13	14	15	16	17	18	19	20	21	22	23	24	25	26	27	28	29	30	31
36.7																																
36.6																																
36.5																																
36.4																																
36.3																																
36.2																																
36.1																																
36.0																																
35.9																																
35.8																																
35.7																																
35.6																																
35.5																																
35.4																																
35.3																																
35.2																																
35.1																																
35.0																																
34.9																																
34.8																																
34.7																																
34.6																																
34.5																																

YOUR REPRODUCTIVE HEALTH

∼

To have healthy hormones we need to remove the chemicals from our personal care products, detergents, packaging, pharmaceuticals, food products and textiles as a starting point. Take the time to look around your bathroom and home and remove the toxic overload. *(See Table 5 on page 57.)*

For our hormones (endocrine system), to be in balance they must support each other and through a thermostat like control mechanism continue to keep your body in balance on a minute by minute day to day basis. Dr Pamela Wartian Smith[3] suggests that for optimal health this system must be in balance throughout your life. As our health agencies are coming to the crossroads of how to help people, together with a greater availability of information, the questions are being asked as to what is causing the problem. In my case, rather than just treating the skin, I have found that there is a deeper problem that lies behind skin conditions such as acne, rosacea and other skin conditions such as psoriasis and atopic dermatitis. The harmony of your hormonal health relies on the relationship of your brain, ovaries/testes/thyroid and adrenals. From your oestrogen and progesterone balance that allows for your normal menstrual cycle, to the balance of testosterone within that cycle, whether you are male or female, we all make these hormones in different amounts and it is this fine and delicate balance that keeps our skin and body healthy and functioning at optimum.

Some of the main factors that affect your hormonal health are:

- contraceptive pill
- hormone replacement therapy (HRT)
- nutrient deficiency, such as vitamins D, A and B complex, Iodine and zinc

- chemical toxicity via xenoestrogens, such as personal care, shampoos, conditioners and cleaning products
- hair colouring with ammonia and processing chemicals
- artificial nails that use polymers and liquid monomer (for example, ethyl methacrylate)
- body-building products, especially those containing D-aspartic acid, whey and other artificial hormonal stimulants.

The female hormonal cycle

In order for a woman to experience optimal health, her body needs to be producing the right balance of hormones at the right time. Oestrogen levels continually rise from the first day of the menstrual cycle and then drop sharply between days 12 and 14 in preparation for ovulation. Following ovulation (when the egg is released — often on day 15), oestrogen remains low whilst the other reproductive hormone, progesterone, rises rapidly during the second half to support fertilisation should this occur. If not progesterone subsequently drops towards the end of the 28-day cycle, to allow for the release and removal of the uterine lining.

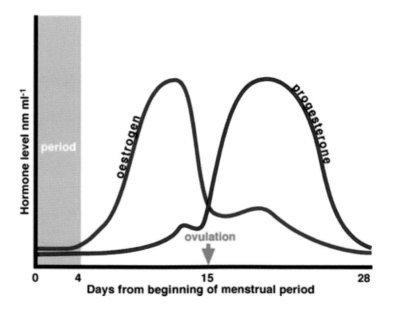

Figure 4: Your reproductive hormones in relation to the days in your menstrual cycle

The female hormonal cycle can be easily upset in our modern world where external sources of oestrogen are sneaking into the body undetected. Our food, especially industrially produced fruits and vegetables, are laden with herbicides and pesticides routinely sprayed on crops and petrochemical residues, called xenoestrogens, from the plastics they are packed in. These compounds have oestrogen-mimicking effects and disrupt the fragile balance of our hormones, abnormally boosting oestrogen levels. Many women also take the contraceptive pill, some without a full understanding of how it prevents pregnancy. The most commonly used types function by elevating oestrogen levels for the first 21 days of the menstrual cycle. This assures oestrogen remains elevated, particularly during the third week of the cycle, the crucial time when fertilisation can take place. Without the drop in oestrogen and elevation of progesterone following conception the egg will not become implanted in the uterus and is flushed out. The problem is that if you are breaking out, especially at this time or your skin rash appears worse, **we know that there is the possibility that your thyroid is also being suppressed by excess oestrogen**. Some studies have shown that plant sources of phytoestrogens, the most potent coming from soy, can cause hormonal disruption and have the potential to cause infertility, hypothyroidism and even breast cancer. This is often due to low iodine levels as iodine is need for healthy detoxification and processing foods containing soy.[14] Chronically high levels of oestrogen in the blood may go unnoticed because the symptoms are not always recognised as being related. These symptoms include:

- premenstrual tension (PMT)
- heavy or irregular bleeding
- fluid retention
- weight gain, particularly around the hips, buttock and thighs
- aggravation of asthma and allergies
- mood swings and bouts of depression
- endometriosis.

If you are experiencing any of the above symptoms, to take control of this problem, your food choices should be focused on balancing oestrogen levels through an increase in non-carbohydrate fibre *(see Table 3 on page 52 for sources of inulin)*, foods that support the detoxification pathways of excess oestrogen via the liver and a reduction in the use of personal care products that contain xenoestrogens or mimic oestrogen. *(See table 5: chemicals to avoid page 57.)*

A successful dietary approach will encourage the reduction of typical food cravings that create further imbalance, such as coffee, tea, alcohol, chocolate and refined sugars. Cruciferous vegetables like broccoli, cauliflower, cabbage and brussels sprouts contain nutrients that help to block the damaging oestrogen detoxification pathway and support the beneficial pathway *(see Table 3 on page 52)*.

However, remember that excess consumption of these vegetables may also require you to include more iodine in your diet. These foods, when part of your weekly programme, together with vitamins A, E and B6, B2, B3 calcium, magnesium and essential fatty acids will support your hormonal health and endocrine system balance.[3,34]

For best results, obtain your food from reliable, naturally grown or reared and organic produce so as to guarantee no detrimental pesticides or petrochemical residues that will increase excess oestrogens. These natural foods will support the body to correctly regulate oestrogen and allow the ebb and flow of your 28-day reproductive cycle. Fluid retention will ease and an appropriate body fat level will more easily be obtained. Daily moods will also become more stable across the month, which will lead to a happier, healthier you!

Table 3: Nutrients and their functions for good health

Nutrient	Functions	Good sources
Vitamin A	Reduces PMT symptoms Supports hormonal conversions	Natural cod liver oil, liver Grass-fed butter, organic, free range eggs
Vitamin B6	Natural diuretic — reduces bloating Contributes to oestrogen regulation	Brown rice Wholewheat, liver, lentils
Vitamin E	Reduces breast tenderness Regulates hormone levels Reduces moodiness and depression	Wheatgerm Wholewheat Raw nuts, olive oil
Calcium	Reduces stress Reduces tension and cramps	Raw milk and cheese Bone broth or stocks, sardines
Magnesium	Reduces stress Reduces tension and cramps	Grass-fed beef, bananas Molasses, dark-green, leafy vegetables
Indole-3-carbinol	Anti-oxidant, blocks oestrogen receptors sites and supports oestrogen elimination from your body	Broccoli, cabbage, cauliflower, kale, brussels sprouts
Inulin	Inulin may facilitate the growth of bifidobacterium within the large Intestine and enhance the production of butyric acid in the colon, which supports colon health and elimination	Banana, wheat, rye, barley, burdock, chicory, dandelion, echinacea, globe artichoke, Jerusalem artichoke, onion, garlic, leek, psyllium
EFAs	Reduces inflammation Supports growing foetus Supports lactation Reduces PMT symptoms	Ocean-caught salmon and tuna Natural cod liver oil Organic, free range eggs Cold-pressed flaxseed oil Evening primrose oil

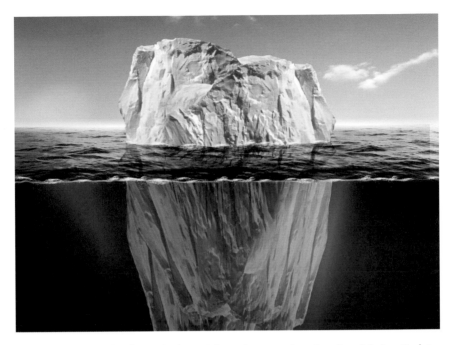

Your combined adrenal, thyroid and reproductive health is vital to your skin and overall health. Without this balance, the body is left exposed to major skin and health issues. Like an iceberg that sits at the bottom of the sea, it is not until it peaks up out of the water that it becomes a problem. This is the same for your hormones as the imbalances are accumulative over time. These imbalances affect the skin's natural defence mechanism (pH), NMF and under- or over-secretion of oil from your sebaceous gland, causing a myriad or symptoms.

Oestrogen dominance questionnaire

Do you have too much or too little oestrogen? We all need to have a balance of hormones and often when our bodies are stressed through diet and lifestyle; our hormones bear the brunt of our actions. Your digestive health also plays a very important role in oestrogen metabolism. With a healthy metabolism requiring a balance of good and bad bacteria (85/15%), a healthy function liver, minimal chemical toxicity such as bromide and an efficient absorption of nutrients.

Check the list and tick the boxes in Table 4 (page 54) to see if your oestrogen level is healthy.

Table 4: Oestrogen dominance questionnaire

Symptoms of oestrogen deficiency

- ☐ Acne
- ☐ Anxiety
- ☐ Arthritis
- ☐ Bladder problems (infections, urinary leakage)
- ☐ Brittle nails and hair
- ☐ Chronic fatigue syndrome
- ☐ Decrease in breast size
- ☐ Decrease in dexterity
- ☐ Decrease in memory
- ☐ Decrease in sexual interest/function
- ☐ Depression
- ☐ Diabetes
- ☐ Dry eyes
- ☐ Elevated blood pressure
- ☐ Elevated cholesterol
- ☐ Food cravings
- ☐ Heart attacks
- ☐ Increase in facial hair
- ☐ Increase in insulin resistance
- ☐ Increase in tension headaches
- ☐ Infertility
- ☐ Low energy, especially at the end of the day
- ☐ Joint pain
- ☐ More frequent migraines
- ☐ More wrinkles — ageing skin
- ☐ Oily skin
- ☐ Osteoporosis
- ☐ Panic attacks
- ☐ Polycystic ovarian syndrome

☐ Restless sleep

☐ Stress incontinence

☐ Strokes

☐ Thinner skin

☐ Thinning hair

☐ Urinary tract infections

☐ Vaginal dryness

☐ Weight gain around the middle

Symptoms of excess oestrogen

☐ Bloating

☐ Decreased sexual interest

☐ Depression with anxiety or agitation

☐ Elevated risk of developing breast cancer

☐ Fatigue

☐ Fibrocystic breasts

☐ Headaches

☐ Heavy periods

☐ Hypothyroidism

☐ Increased risk of autoimmune disease

☐ Increased risk of developing uterine cancer

☐ Irritability

☐ Mood swings

☐ Panic attacks

☐ Swollen breasts

☐ Uterine fibroids

☐ Water retention

☐ Weight gain, especially around the abdomen, hips and thighs.

> *Please note:*
>
> *Your stress hormones, cortisol and adrenaline; sex hormones, progesterone, oestrogen, testosterone and pregnenolone; and metabolic hormones, insulin and thyroxine, are all part of your healthy hormone balance. We have briefly focused on your oestrogen/reproductive hormone health as one of the most common causes of skin conditions starts with hormonal stress, imbalance and sensitivity to medications such as the contraceptive pill.*
>
> *If you suspect you are oestrogen-dominant, it is worthwhile reassessing any medication you are on. If you don't need it, consider eliminating it. Reassess your fibre intake as you can support healthy elimination with the use of plant fibre such as psyllium husks and inulin. (See "Digestive health" on page 59.)*

The oestrogenic effect

To have healthy hormones we also need to reduce the many chemicals that our skin is exposed to in our skin care and personal care products, such as detergents, packaging, pharmaceuticals, food products and textiles. To follow is a short list of **chemicals best to avoid** (there are more being discovered all the time for more information go to www.healthandenvironment.org/tddb) and known hormone disruptors (xenoestrogens), to reduce your exposure and the negative hormonal effects. Remember, this goes hand in hand with the food that you choose to eat to nourish your body and the lifestyle that you lead.

Table 5: Chemicals to avoid

Alkylphenol: Synthetic surfactants used in some detergents and cleaning products.

Atrazine: Weed killer.

4-methlbenzylidene camphor (4-MBC): Ingredients in sunscreens, safe if less than 10% of product.

Brominated flame retardants (BFRs): Widely used in furniture.

Butylated hydroxyanisole (BHA): Food preservative.

Bisphenol-A: Monomer for polycarbonate plastics and epoxy resin; antioxidant in plasticisers used in container liners. (Check that the plastics you are using have a triangle with a number in them — you want at least 2 or higher.)

DDT: Insecticide.

Dichlorodiphenyldichloroethylene and dichlorodiphenyl dichloroethylene dieldrin. By-product of the breakdown of DDT.

Endosulfan: Insecticide.

Erythrosine (E127): Food colouring banned in Norway and USA.

Ethinylestradiol (combined oral contraceptive pill): Released into the environment as a xenoestrogen.

Heptachlor: Insecticide.

Lindane/Hexachlorocyclohexane: Insecticide.

Metallo-oestrogens: A class of inorganic xenoestrogens.

Methoxychlor: Insecticide.

Non-phenol and derivatives: Industrial surfactants, emulsifiers to emulsion polymerisation, laboratory detergents, pesticides.

Polychlorinated biphenyls (PCBs): In electrical oils, lubricants, adhesives and paints.

Parabens: Lotions, skin care, body care.

Phenosulfonthiazine: A red dye in make-up/clothing/food.

Phthalates (plasticisers) DEHP: Plasticiser for PVC.

Propylgallate: Food additive.

When considering the oestrogen effect in our food there are some foods that are more likely to be contaminated than others. Here are some of the foods that are more highly sprayed and contaminated. Remember to wash your food well before you store it and, where possible, to reduce these contaminants, buy organic or spray-free, or even better grow your own vegies and fruit if you can. There are some great micro garden kits available that cater to most urban spaces, small or large.

Table 6: The highly sprayed and the clean

The highly sprayed (in order of contamination)	The clean (in order of least contamination)
Apples	Onions
Celery	Sweet corn
Capsicum	Pineapples
Peaches	Avocado
Nectarines	Sweet peas
Strawberries	Cabbage
Grapes	Asparagus
Spinach	Mangoes
Lettuce	Eggplant
Cucumbers	Kiwi fruit
Blueberries	Rockmelon
Potatoes	Watermelon
Sweet potatoes	Grapefruit
Mushrooms	

Summary

To reduce your exposure to harmful chemicals that disrupt your hormones and endocrine system through an accumulative effect, choose your skin care products, toothpastes, shampoos, conditioners, washing powders and detergents carefully, where possible, and eat food that is less contaminated without the harmful sprays. Any little change that you implement and maintain will give you cumulative benefits throughout your life!

DIGESTIVE HEALTH

ॐ

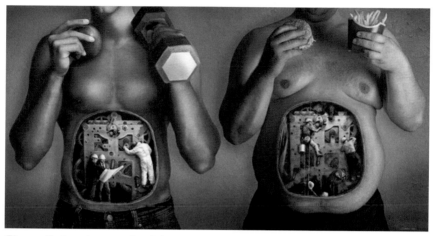

Figure 5: Good versus bad digestive health

A healthy digestion equates to health skin as they are both excretory systems, (they eliminate toxins from your body) and support each other to keep your body clean, healthy and functioning like a "well-oiled" machine. Chuktan[54], 2005, suggest that we should think of our body as a factory. Organs like your lungs, kidneys and liver represent the machinery that keeps the body's production going; extracting oxygen, filtering blood, removing toxins, synthesising hormones and performing lots of complicated tasks to keep us alive. We house our machinery but who tells it what to do? Our microbes do! In fact they are the ones that break down our food, determine who gets absorbed verses who gets eliminated. They help distinguish between real infection and colonisation of harmless bacteria and tell our immune system when to rally and when to relax. We have evolved over millions of years to host an incredible army of microbes that produce substances our bodies cannot make and fight our battles for us. They can even turn our genes on and off. So it is important to understand our digestive tract and how we can support out microbes in their plight to keep us happy and healthy.

Summary of your Microbial family and how they assist you[54]

- Convert sugars to short chain fatty acids for energy

- Crowds out harmful bacteria

- Digests the food you eat

- Assists your body to absorb nutrients such as calcium and iron

- Supports a healthy pH (You can monitor this daily by testing your urine)

- Supports and maintains the healthy lining and integrity of your digestive tract

- Metabolises/breakdown drugs

- Modulates your genes

- Neutralises cancer causing compounds

- Produces your digestive enzymes

- Synthesise B Complex (Thiamine, folate & pyridoxine) and Fat Soluable vitamins (Such as Vitamin K)

- Synthesises hormones (a very important task to get right for healthy skin).

- Trains the immune system to distinguish friend from foe

Your digestive tract consists of

- your mouth and salivary glands, this is where digestion starts.

- your oesophagus – the tube that takes your food to the stomach.

- your stomach this is where your food is manipulated and broken down using gastric enzymes, hydrochloric acid and movement, called peristalsis, to further break down the food.

- Your small intestines – This is where some of the many trillions of microbes live in your digestive tract and each species and colony have a job to do to assist you in further break down of the food you eat to give you the end result of vitamins, minerals, amino acids (breakdown from protein), sugars and fats. Now your body has some fuel!

- Your pancreas – responsible for sugar balance by the release of insulin as well as pancreatic enzymes that support the breakdown of the food you eat.

- Your liver – Our liver performs many essential functions related to digestion, metabolism, immunity, and the storage of nutrients within the body. These functions make the liver a vital organ without which the tissues of the body would quickly die from lack of energy and nutrients. Everything that you eat, drink, inhale, ingest, and absorb through your skin passes through your liver via your blood.

- Your gallbladder – Bile is a mixture of water, bile salts, cholesterol, and the pigment bilirubin that is made by the cells in your liver and concentrated and stored in your gallbladder. As you eat bile travels through the bile ducts and is released into your small intestine where it emulsifies large masses of fat. The emulsification of fats by bile turns the large clumps of fat into smaller pieces that have more surface area and are therefore easier for your body to digest. Research has shown that a healthy gallbladder completes a healthy digestive track and also supports the healthy microflora.

- Your appendix – 30 years ago your appendix was not considered to have any real value in your health and thought to be a leftover of our ancestors. However we now know that your appendix is very important as it acts as a reservoir for your microflora and is released in times of stress and infection to support colon health and elimination.

- Your colon – The function of your large intestine is to remove food leftovers after the nutrients have been removed from it together with bacteria and other waste. This process is called peristalsis and can take around 36 hours depending on the health of your digestive tract. It is very important to be aware of how your stool should be at the end process of digestion because this will tell you if you are absorbing your nutrients, eliminating toxins and well hydrated. I guess this is the time where we do a little toilet talk and I like to educate my clients so that they know how to monitor their health on a day to day basis. If your are healthy your stool or poo will look like type 3 or 4 of the **Bristol Stool Chart** (see Figure 6) and you should be able to eliminate easily at least once a day. The size of your stools indicates the health of your beneficial digestive microbes. So, generally speaking, the larger the stool the better and more diverse your microbes are which loosely translates into a happier healthy gut.[53]

• anus – the exit point.

Figure 6 Bristol Stool Chart

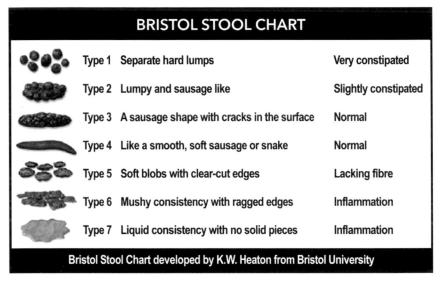

BRISTOL STOOL CHART		
Type 1	Separate hard lumps	Very constipated
Type 2	Lumpy and sausage like	Slightly constipated
Type 3	A sausage shape with cracks in the surface	Normal
Type 4	Like a smooth, soft sausage or snake	Normal
Type 5	Soft blobs with clear-cut edges	Lacking fibre
Type 6	Mushy consistency with ragged edges	Inflammation
Type 7	Liquid consistency with no solid pieces	Inflammation

Bristol Stool Chart developed by K.W. Heaton from Bristol University

Your digestive tract is vital to your health as I am sure you're now starting to fully understand. It is a complete tube or pipe, so to speak, from your mouth to your anus (see figure 7 page 65). There are many things that can affect both the health and the efficiency of your digestive tract that can then result in your digestive tract becoming more porous or the functional medical term is **"dysbosis."**

Dysbosis is an alteration of the microbial community and we will talk a little more about dysbosis later. (See page 63). As you have seen previously your microbial family is very important to maintain so many areas of your health, hormones, nutrition and skin. If there is an ongoing imbalances/problem the body will start to tell you this in the way of sign and symptoms. You might like to go through the checklist below to see how healthy your microbial family. If you have more than one of these symptoms a review of your cooking habits and what you eat as well as adding a probiotic, (further information on probiotics later in this section), and fermented food and drink to your diet is essential to help your body recolonise. You can check your progress by monitoring your pH.

Do you have the symptoms of digestive tract dysbosis?

☐ Acne, eczema and rosacea

☐ Allergies and chronic food sensitivities

☐ Bad breath and gum disease

☐ Bloating or foul smelling gas

☐ Brain fog

☐ Poor sleep or insomnia

☐ Candida overgrowth or chronic yeast infection

☐ Long term unexplained fatigue

☐ Depression or anxiety

☐ Difficulty in losing weight

☐ Frequent colds/flues/or sinus infections

☐ Mucus in your stools or regular loose stools

☐ Poor digestion such as reflux, sugar cravings, tiredness after meals

☐ Stomach Bugs or episodes of food poisoning

☐ Unexplained diarrhoea

☐ Vaginal or anal itching

The risk factors that promote dysbosis are:

✓ Regular or consistent mental, physical or emotional stress.

✓ Dehydration as your body is 70% water and needs to be hydrated to break down your food.

✓ Low nutritional value of food eaten therefore there are less nutrients that can be broken down for absorption and use.

- ✓ Excessive consumption of foods containing hydrogenated fats such as pastries, cakes, biscuits, burgers, chips and ice-cream.[52] (As they block our healthy fats, such as advocado, from completing their tasks and as a result this affects the healthy communicate between our immune system and our intestinal microbes in our small intestine.

- ✓ Ingestion of alcohol especially without food i.e. a meal[52]

- ✓ Regular use of off the shelf medications and prescriptions as they affect the numbers of healthy microbes such as antibiotics, reflux medication, contraceptive pill & steroids and nonsteroidal inflammatory such as aspirin medication.[53]

- ✓ Inadequate ingestion of daily fibre as not enough fibre can be even worse for your microbiome than high ingestion of sugar, starches and fats. The recommended amount of daily fibre is 25-35grams per day that is in a non processed form. Certain types of dietary fibre are needed to detoxification and eliminate fat soluble toxins & excess hormones.

- ✓ Removal or your appendix – as your microbial reservoir has now been removed.

- ✓ Regular use of hand sanitisers – As our healthy bodies are colonised with many different microbes that are good for us. When you continually scrub them away or chemically remove them you are doing more harm than good. Like the over use of antibiotics if you are obsessed with sanitisers you will be knocking out important species that sometimes never fully recover leading to a less diverse and more fragile microbiome. The use of soap water and friction (rubbing your hands together), is the best method of keeping yourself healthy.

- ✓ Drinking chlorinated water

- ✓ Artificial sweeteners

- ✓ Ingesting too much sugar and fat as in a processed, fast food diet.

- ✓ Infections

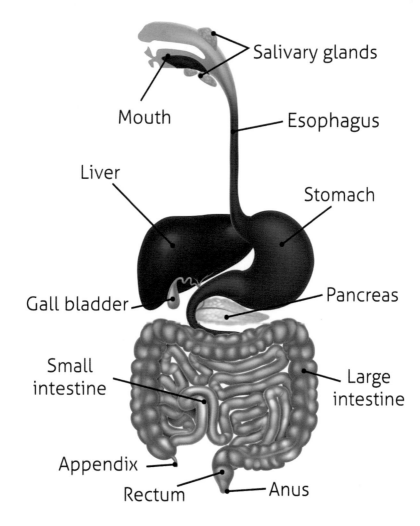

Figure 7 Your digestive tract

Digestive health check at a glance

We all now know how important our skin health relies on a healthy digestion and its family of microbiome. But how do you know, on a daily basis if your digestion is happy and your choices and changes are making a difference.

Here's an easy test, based on traditional Chinese medicine, that you can use to check your health. When your digestion is healthy your tongue looks healthy too and is generally a good pinkish colour all over. However when the colour of your tongue changes this is highly representative of digestive problems.

Stand in front of a mirror and poke out your tongue what do you see? If you see a coating on your tongue which can range from white to a yellow or brown shade, then you are looking at an imbalance of digestive flora. The Chinese interpret problems by checking the sides of the tongue which indicate liver health. The tip of the tongue represents the stomach and the front of the tongue represents the upper intestine and the back of the tongue as the large intestine or colon. In reality this usually proves to be absolutely correct and many people with a Candida infection will find either the front and, more usually, the back of the tongue are coated and discoloured. If this is you then it is most certainly worth your while getting checked out for Candida overgrowth and it may be the reason you are experiencing your skin problem.

Probiotics and how they can help you return to a healthy balance

You may now be having a light bulb moment and beginning to understand more completely the relationship between your digestive tract, your health, your skin and your microbiome family. In fact some researchers believe that our microbiome is as individual as we are and as such as like our fingerprint – unique to us[52, 53].

As we have discussed previously our microbiome maintain and have an effect all areas of our body. Low energy production and vitality was once more isolated and accepted as " just aging," but now we have proof that stress, diet, sleep deprivation, hormonal deficiencies, chronic infections and nutritional deficiencies play a significant role in depleting our vital spark at any age and as a result chronic infections, hormonal imbalances, obesity, acne, rosacea are the signs and symptoms. Now what do these symptoms have in common – they all also reflect a dysbosis! (*Go to page 63 for signs and symptoms*).

One of the discoveries that I was interested in, as I am often asked the question; " why can't food alone help us recovery from illness?" I had to ask and then research – Is it that our genetic differences affect our ability to obtain and absorb optimal levels of various nutrients from our diet even when it is nutritionally dense or is it that our medical history is encased in regular use of antibiotics, medications and being born C Section? My research brought me back to digestive health and your microbiome family. In some cases people that have experienced a lot of illness as a child or self medicated, without realising it have slowly reduced their diverse family of microbiome and it is this loss that creates the symptoms of poor health, skin conditions and disease.[52,53,54]

Clinical note:

*I now understand, from my own medical background, why I had acne and chronic health problems. In a nutshell I was given strong antibiotics as a baby (That's one hit for the poor developing microbiome). I was a picky kid and not good with food suffering anxiety and depression from as early as 10 years. Once I got into my adolescence years I had a lot of medical problems which resulted in lots of medication, antibiotics, and medical intervention. Again my microbiome would have struggled to maintain their healthy numbers being constantly supressed due to the effects of the medication. In my thirties I went through a very challenging time with my health and suffered extreme energy loss, insomnia, hormonal imbalances, hot flushes, breast lumps and so on – needless to say it was not a fun time. What I want to share with you is that **what we now know** about our digestive tract was not know 30 years ago and it is only now that we are starting to understand the importance of our gut flora and how it impacts our health, our life, our wellness. So this is always an important area to address when treating skin conditions however it needs to be the right one!*

Whether the medications are off the shelf or prescribed, the impact of medications and their regular use into our health culture is now being more understood as well as the impacts that it is having on us.

Ten years ago it was not so common to take probiotics whilst on antibiotics however now, I am pleased to say, it is common place, as you are more likely to understand the implications on your digestive health. Whether you are taking the contraceptive pill, hay fever medication, anti inflammatory or indigestion medication they will all have an impact on your digestive health affecting it's microbiome and as a result its effectiveness, efficiency and therefore your available vitamins, minerals, proteins and good fats that available to power your body. Therefore anyone who is taking any medication, in my clinical opinion, should be also taking a broad spectrum probiotic.

I would suggest Lactobacillis or Bifidobacteria microbiome families for anyone that is taking the contraceptive pill, indigestion tablets or any regular medications. If you are on long term antibiotics the beneficial bacteria of choice is Saccaromyces boulardii[55] as this strain has been shown to be resistant to all antibiotics and therefore able to ward off potential and harmful gut imbalances or dysbosis caused by the antibiotic.

> **In a nutshell: The food you eat + the conversion of that food = the benefits for you all rely on your unique balance of microbiome, health and vitality. However one thing that will always change the rules to the equation is synthetic medication in which you would be best to add daily probiotic support.**

However you can also support your digestive tract and microbiome family in other way such as adding kefir and fermented foods to your diet.

The link between your digestive health, your fibre intake, and your skin is essential to understand, just as important as your microbiome family that we discussed earlier. A diet low in grains and fibre reduces your body's ability to metabolise excess hormones such as oestrogen through poor elimination and a slow and congested digestive system — a bit like a traffic jam. Add in other factors such as the contraceptive pill, HRT, environmental oestrogen or xeno-oestrogens such as parabens and petrochemicals *(ingredients in our personal care and home care products that we use and absorb on a daily basis through our skin)*, lack of exercise and increased daily stress on the body from our high-paced modern life, and you have a recipe for high levels of hormones to be retained by your body that will cause havoc to your hormonal health, your digestive health and your skin.[3,12,25]

Daily consumption of fibre such as inulin, psyllium, wheat bran and larch is essential for a healthy digestive function, not only because it supports elimination and detoxification but also because it supports another vital function in the digestive tract, the production of a short-chain fatty acid called butyric acid. **Butyric acid** acts as a nutrient for the beneficial bacteria within your digestive tract that help keep your digestive process moving, which, in turn, results in a healthy and efficient digestive tract *(see Table 3 on page 52 for food examples)*.

To help you gain a clearer picture, imagine the processing plants in your digestive tract and every time you eat your body is processing the foods that you eat and breaking them down, with the help of your microbiome, into small packets of fuel (glucose), to support and repair your body. It stands to reason, then, that if the food that you eat is already processed there is little fuel left that can be extracted for your health.[1]

There is little doubt that the modern processed diet, high in daily alcohol, sugars and fats and low in fibre and nutrition, wreaks havoc with your digestive health and, in turn, the health of your skin. So let's discuss this a little further to show why the choices that you make have the impact that they do.

One aspect of the Western, quick-fix, ready-to-go meals is that it disrupts the sensitive balance of your beneficial microbiome, causes inflammation of your digestive tract and disturbs the gut-associated immune system causing **dysbiosis**.

The term dysbiosis was originally introduced in the early 1900s by Dr Eli Metchnikoff to describe an imbalance of the bacteria in the gut. Literally it means "dys" incorrect and "biosis" life. The word comes from "symbiosis", meaning to reside together harmoniously, with dysbiosis meaning the opposite. He coined the expression that "Death begins in the gut!". Metchnikoff was awarded the Nobel Prize in 1908 for his work on friendly bacterial flora.[38] He introduced the idea that fermented milk products (at that time unpasteurised and unhomogenised) could prove beneficial to the gut, inhibiting bacterial infection. He believed that the root of many diseases was via intestinal bacteria decomposing protein in the bowel. Lactic acid-producing bacteria were believed to stunt the production of the pathogenic/disease causing bacteria.[1]

Beta-glucuronidase is a carcinogen made within the digestive tract in a state of dysbosis[37] and it **interferes with the liver's ability to break down and therefore eliminate excess oestrogen**[5], thereby contributing to oestrogen dominance which may also be amplified with low iodine levels. Butyric acid, feeds and nourishes the digestive tract, including the beneficial bacteria, which are responsible for beneficial fermentation. Without this source of fuel, the digestive tract is more likely to become inflamed and the balance of beneficial (85%) to detrimental bacteria (15%) difficult to achieve.

Other ways to support digestive health and maintain the delicate balance is by using kefir milk or coconut water or yoghurt daily, **because kefir not only supports the production of more beneficial bacteria but also the manufacture of butyric acid, which we know is beneficial to our digestive health, which over time flows onto our skin by recolonising our digestive tract microbiome.**

What is kefir?

The word "kefir" is derived from the Turkish word *keif*, which literally translates to the "good feeling" one has after drinking it.[38] Traditional cultures have attributed healing powers to kefir for centuries, but it has only recently become the subject of scientific research to determine its true therapeutic value.

Traditionally, kefir is a fermented milk product that originated centuries ago in the Caucasus Mountains, and is now enjoyed by many different cultures worldwide, particularly in Europe and Asia. It can be made from the milk of any ruminant animal, such as a cow, goat or sheep or from seeds, beans and even water. It is slightly sour and carbonated due to the fermentation activity of the symbiotic colony of bacteria and yeast that make up the "grains" used to culture the milk (not actual grains, but a grain-like matrix of proteins, lipids and sugars that feed the microbes). The various types of beneficial microbiota contained in kefir make it one of the most potent probiotic foods available *(see Table 7 on page 71)*.

Besides containing highly beneficial bacteria and yeasts, kefir is a rich source of many different vitamins, minerals and essential amino acids that promote healing and repair, as well as general health maintenance.[38] Kefir contains high levels of thiamine, B12, calcium, folate and vitamin K2. It is a good source of biotin, a B vitamin that helps the body assimilate other B vitamins. This is particularly beneficial when you are low in iodine as you need B2 and B3 to absorb and support Iodine uptake. (Remember that iodine is essential for a healthy metabolism, detoxification and thyroid.) The complete proteins in kefir are already partially digested, and are therefore more easily utilised by the body. Like many other dairy products, kefir is a great source of minerals such as calcium and magnesium, as well as phosphorus, which helps the body utilise carbohydrates, fats and proteins for cell growth, maintenance and energy.

Kefir grains are a combination of lactic acid bacteria and yeasts in a matrix of proteins, lipids and sugars, and this symbiotic matrix (or SCOBY) forms "grains" that resemble cauliflower. For this reason, a complex and highly variable community of lactic acid bacteria and yeasts can be found in these grains, although some are predominant; *Lactobacillus* species are always present.

Table 7: The beneficial bacteria, yeast, vitamins and minerals in a general kefir product

Beneficial bacteria	Beneficial yeast
Lactobacillus acidophilus	*Candida humilis*
Lactobacillus brevis	*Kazachstania unispora*
Lactobacillus casei	*Kazachstania exigua*
Lactobacillus delbrueckii subsp. *bulgaricus*	*Kluyveromyces siamensis*
Lactobacillus sake	*Kluyveromyces lactis*
Lactobacillus delbrueckii subsp. *delbrueckii*	*Kluyveromyces marxianus*
Lactobacillus delbrueckii subsp. *lactis*	*Saccharomyces cerevisiae*
Lactobacillus helveticus	*Saccharomyces unisporus*
Lactobacillus kefiranofaciens subsp. kefiranofaciens	**Plus vitamins**
Lactobacillus kefiri	Vitamin A
Lactobacillus paracasei subsp. *paracasei*	Vitamin B1
Lactobacillus plantarum	Vitamin B2
Lactobacillus rhamnosus	Vitamin B6

table continued next page

Beneficial bacteria	Beneficial yeast
Lactococcus lactis subsp. *cremoris*	Vitamin D
Lactococcus lactis subsp. *lactis*	Vitamin K2
Lactococcus lactis	Folic acid
Leuconostoc mesenteroides subsp. *cremoris*	Nicotinic acid
Leuconostoc mesenteroides subsp.*dextranicum*	
Leuconostoc mesenteroides subsp. *mesenteroides*	**Plus minerals**
Pseudomonas	Calcium
Pseudomonas fluorescens	Iron
Pseudomonas putida	Iodine
Saccharomyces martiniae	
Streptococcus thermophilus	**And water**

Diet and lifestyle

The most important kick-starts to immediately boost your skin's health are based in your daily habits, the changes that you implement and the consistency in your approach. A helpful way to keep you on track, I find, is by keeping a diary. Take time to think about the things that you do on a daily basis, such as that cup of coffee first thing in the morning, going to work without any breakfast, working all day and not drinking water, or ruminating over things that are out of your control.

I know it sounds like a cliché and I am sure that you have heard it many times before, but you are the result of an accumulation of your habits: to take the stairs or not take the stairs, what you eat and drink, and the relationships that you have with your food, family, loved ones, work colleagues and yourself.

It takes 30 days to change a habit, so if you are ready for the change you need to make sure that you stay on track for at least 30 days!

If you feel as though you are ready for a change, to follow are a few things you can implement immediately.

1. Eliminate dairy, milk, butter, cheese, yoghurt, cream, ice cream. *(See "Dairy and its effect on skin" on page 86)*

2. Eliminate or change the amount of sugar intake you eat on a daily basis to natural sugars such as agave, coconut sugar, stevia, xylitol, and raw honey. Make it your goal to reduce your total processed sugar intake down to 3 grams a day but do be aware that fruit juices are rich in concentrated fructose and can overload your body in a similar way to sugar.

3. Eliminate all processed, fast food and long life foods from your diet. They have little to no nutritional benefit in your diet and the health of your skin and hormones. Plus a lot of the pastries, pastas and breads contain bromide, which results in iodine deficiency and a sluggish, unhappy thyroid equals a sluggish, unhappy you!

4. Drink 1–1.5 litres filtered water a day (make sure it is fluoride and chloride free, as the halogen fluoride also blocks the thyroid receptors in the same way as bromide and chloride. This results in an unhappy, sluggish thyroid). To increase hydration and taste, why not add a dash of fresh lemon juice.

Clinical note:

I have found with the clients that I am treating if they have problems with their nutrition and it is out of balance, with low levels of vitamin D, zinc, B12, iodine, and vitamin K, drinking water half an hour before meals rather than at meals results in fewer digestive problems such as reflux, bloating and tiredness after meals.

Often too much water at meal times will dilute your digestive enzymes and make digestion sluggish, especially if you are low in your digestive enzymes, iodine and stomach acids: hydrochloric acid. Once your levels are back to normal it doesn't seem to be such a problem.

---

5. Add 1–2 tablespoons raw, unfiltered apple cider vinegar to 100 ml water and sip with your meals if you feel you are slow and sluggish and your temperature is constantly below 36.0° Celsius or 96.8° Fahrenheit. *(See the information on basal metabolic temperature and thyroid health on page 47.)*

6. Reduce your coffee, eliminate carbonated and energy drinks, reduce alcohol intake and have it as a treat rather than daily.

The dos and don'ts of healthy skin

Table 8: The dos and don'ts of healthy skin

Don't
Eat too many raisins, bananas, dates and grapes as they contain fast-releasing sugars. Instead choose apples, apricots, blackberries, cherries, grapefruit, lemons, limes, nectarines, peaches, pears, raspberries, strawberries and watermelon.
Ruminate and over think problems that lead to mental stress and anguish. Trust in yourself and your ability to problem solve. Have a trusted friend as a sounding board rather than a judgement maker.
Drink soft drinks, sports drinks and dairy-laden packaged drinks, chocolate milk and hot chocolate.
Eat highly processed foods as they will rapidly increase your blood sugar level.
Be unprepared with your meals. A healthy diet takes time to prepare. You need to plan, shop and cook.
Use petrochemical-based products such as PEG, propylene glycol, betanite, clay and Camphor methylbenzene above 10 mg or any of the benzenes on your skin — they are skin irritants. They are known to strip the skin of moisture and destabilise your skin's pH and hormonal health (oestrogen dominance).
Expect your new skin care regime to heal your skin in 1 or 2 days. It will take time for your skin to heal and the lifestyle changes to take affect. Allow at least 30 days before reassessing your results.
Go to bed late on a regular basis and get up early. Contrary to popular belief, your body needs eight hours to rest and recuperate from the day-to-day stressors.
Use alcohol based mouthwashes as they can destroy the microbial ecosystem in your mouth.
Use hand sanitizers.

Do

Eat foods such as broccoli, green beans, carrots, long and brown rice, wholegrains, such as quinoa and barley, to add more fibre to your diet.

If you are experiencing bloating or digestive symptoms, try 1–2 tablespoons in 100 ml water of fermented apple cider vinegar with your meals to support digestion. Sip during meals, check your iodine levels and add kefir to your daily routine.

Eliminate any dairy-based foods such as milk, cream, yoghurt, cheese, butter. They increase the insulin growth factor and contribute to all skin conditions, especially acne, by irritating the sebaceous gland and increasing blood sugar levels and growing more pimples!

Exercise daily for at least 30 minutes. Interval training is best for those with insulin resistance *(see questionnaire).*

Avoid or reduce your alcohol intake or have at least 2 alcohol free days.

Take a quality omega-3 supplement and eat fish preferably wild such as salmon, mackerel, tuna, herring and sardines three times a week.

Also good plant sources are chia, pumpkin seeds and walnuts.

Use nutritious topical skin products that support the normal pH of 4.5–5.5, reduce inflammation and rebalance moisture.

Add kefir yoghurt, water and drinks to your diet. They are great at rebalancing the health of your digestive tract. *(See "Digestive health" on page 59.)*

Take a broad spectrum probiotic if your are taking medication or craving sugars during the day or in times of stress. I find that the probiotic Saccharomyces boulardii twice a day works well for most people.

Oil pulling

You might find this hard to believe as it is such a simple, yet powerful therapy, but oral cleansing has a powerful benefit to your skin condition and has been around for over 2000 years. Why haven't you heard about it? Good question, as it is so simple and that's maybe why it gets passed over ...

Oil pulling comes from the wisdom of Ayurvedic medicine, the link between oral hygiene/health and skin complaints, as well as chronic conditions, is well known and researched.[44] In fact, if you have or have had bleeding gums, have had root canal treatment or any other poor dental health problems you will be bound to have other issues of bacterial overgrowth in your mouth — the start of your digestive tract. Some other health complaints are migraine headaches, asthma, diabetes, chronic fatigue, rash of unknown origins, chronic allergies or sinusitis, and the list goes on.

Whilst most people may say, "But I regularly brush and floss", the cold, hard facts are that 90% of the population has some degree of gum disease or tooth decay.[44]

Just as the eyes are viewed as the window to the soul, the mouth is the window to the digestive system, and when you look inside your mouth you see a representation of the condition of your entire intestinal tract. The bacteria and other microorganisms that inhibit our mouths influence our health and skin. Inside your mouth, the cells are replacing themselves every three to seven days and the bacteria in the mouth fall into two categories:

1. Planktonic or free-floating, which is found in the saliva; and

2. Biofilm — the bacteria that colonise on the surfaces of the mouth such as the teeth and tongue.

Your mouth harbours over 600 types of bacteria and the amount of bacteria is estimated to be around 10 billion. Anaerobic bacteria produce enzymes and toxins as by-products, which damage and irritate the gums, causing inflammation and bleeding. When you brush you are only reaching 60% of the surfaces of your teeth, leaving plaque in hard-to-reach places such as in between the teeth.

Your mouth, teeth and gums are abundant with blood supply and so it is very easy for bacteria to invade your body and affect other areas of your health. In fact, research has shown that, should you have a pet dog, your dog's mouth will be cleaner than your partner's, parents', and others.[44] Why? Dogs have antibodies in their saliva that are not found in humans and it is these antibodies that kill disease-causing germs!

So, now that I have explained a little about this, I hope that you are chomping at the bit, so to speak, to start moving towards beautiful, healthy skin and a healthy digestive system to match.

So how do I do It? The therapy or technique is called "oil pulling" and it is very simple.

1. Choose oil that you have in your pantry/cupboard, such as coconut oil, sesame seed, sunflower, macadamia, apricot kernel and so on — you can't make a wrong choice; it's personal preference. I like macadamia oil myself.

2. Starting on an empty stomach — you might want to drink some water beforehand if your mouth feels dry.

3. Take 2–3 teaspoons of liquid oil in your mouth and start sucking, pushing, pulling the oil through your teeth, around your mouth and through and around your gums. **Do not gargle the oil.**

4. Continue for 15–20 minutes. I like to be time-effective as I do this so I also, at the same time, I get ready for work, check my emails, and so on.

5. As you move the oil around your mouth during the next 15–20 minutes it will turn into a milky-white fluid. Once you have completed this process, discard the oil in the rubbish bin.

6. Rinse out your mouth and have a drink of water.

7. Follow this procedure at least once a day, but two to three times a day if you have acne, rosacea, atopic dermatitis, psoriasis, sinusitis, hay fever or any skin condition or chronic illness as they all affect your digestion and its health.

Whilst I make no bones about advocating beautiful, healthy skin through live food that has been minimally processed, sprayed and/or contaminated, daily habitual activity, nutritionally based skin care, exercise and the importance of a good night's sleep are also vitally important. This therapy, in conjunction with those practices, will have you on the road to good skin health.

Clinical note:

I had an acne client who started oil pulling very enthusiastically. She was dedicated to improving her health and skin and so was completing oil pulling twice a day for 20 minutes using macadamia oil. She contacted me a week into the therapy and said that she had developed a rash over her trunk and arms and it was spreading down her legs, so as you can appreciate she was getting very worried. After quizzing her for 10 minutes or so it was obvious that she was not doing anything else that was different, so we agreed that it must be the oil pulling and I advised her to stop the oil pulling to see if the rash changed. Within 24 hours of stopping this therapy her rash had subsided and she was returning to normal!

It highlighted to us both how powerful this therapy is in detoxifying the body and removing toxins, although it doesn't seem like much at the time.

She recommended oil pulling a week later and started doing alternate days and then slowing increased her frequency back to daily but did it slowly over a month, starting with every third day, alternate days and so on. The rash did not return. Interestingly she was also iodine deficient so we started her on potassium iodide and iodine and now she is moving forward in leaps and bounds and oil pulling is a lifelong habit.

Vitamin D

Skin and hormonal health is never complete unless we discuss vitamin D and address any misconceptions. With this thought in mind, a healthy dietary food intake and some sun exposure is a good balance for healthy skin, or so we once thought. I find that many of my clients — nine out of 10 —are vitamin D deficient and significantly so!

Food sources of vitamin D are fish such as tuna, mackerel and salmon, and eggs. It is difficult to ensure the potency of vitamin D supplements if they have not been processed correctly. Therefore, if you need to supplement your intake, purchase a practitioner-quality product and ensure that it is in an opaque container.

Vitamin D is now getting a lot more attention, but when I first started treating people it was very much overlooked. People would come into the clinic with vitamin D levels as low as 17 nmol. This is a very dangerous level, when good skin and hormonal health requires a level of at least 75–100 nmol.[13]

You may not realise that you are deficient in vitamin D as it can only be diagnosed with a blood test. However, some of the symptoms of low vitamin D levels are:

- burning throat and mouth
- cramps
- sleeplessness
- softening of bones and teeth
- irritated digestive system
- skin conditions such as acne and rosacea.

Vitamin D also plays an important role in reducing wrinkles and is often found to be low in skin conditions such as eczema, psoriasis and atopic dermatitis. Even though it is a vitamin, it does behave more like a hormone in our bodies and acts as a powerful anti-oxidant and anti-carcinogenic, which can assist in the prevention of skin cancer together with vitamin A, heart disease and diabetes. It can also help to:

- enhance the absorption of calcium and regulate blood levels of phosphorous
- aid in relief of depression
- assist in maintaining a health immune system
- assist in maintaining healthy wound healing
- assist with sleep disorders and anxiety
- support a healthy thyroid.

The most common source of vitamin D is from the sun. However, due to the increasing rate of diagnosed skin cancers in some countries, people are concerned about too much sun exposure. Australia and New Zealand have the highest incidence and mortality rates of melanoma in the world, according to Australia's Department of Health and Ageing. In these two countries, the risk of developing melanoma before the age of 75 is 1 in 24 for males and 1 in 34 for females.[13]

This has led to a fear about exposing your skin for too long in the sun and due to the increase in the use of sunblock and abstinence from the sun we have increased the incidence of vitamin D deficiency.

In most countries, as everyone's skin type/colour/age is different, I suggest two to three times a week between 10 am and 3 pm that you expose your arms, legs and trunk (for males) to the sun. If you are making vitamin D, just look beside you at your shadow and if it is longer than you are tall you are not making vitamin D but more than likely risking skin damage.

If you want to use the sun rays to make your own vitamin D then your shadow should be the same size or shorter than you are and you will want to stay in the sun until you feel and see your skin go pink — this is called one *erythema dose*. You now need to go into the shade or cover up but leave your skin to cool. Do not shower for at least 20 minutes, as your skin needs time to absorb the sun's rays and make vitamin D.

To assess whether or not you are being successful in having a healthy vitamin D level you should consider a regular annual blood test to ensure that the actions that you have put into place are affective as there are lifestyle factors that require an extra demand for vitamin D.

These factors that demand higher amounts of vitamin D for optimum health are:

- regular alcohol consumption
- a digestive disorder that results in diarrhoea or episodic diarrhoea
- pregnancy and lactation
- medications such as anti-convulsants
- medical conditions such as Crohn's disease, ulcerative colitis, breast or prostatic cancer, diabetes and liver disorders, to name a few.

Whilst there is still no real agreement internationally on the therapeutic dose of vitamin D, in Australia we range from 75–100 nmol.

> *Clinical note:*
>
> *I have had many clients of Asian, Indian and Mediterranean origin, whose results will come back as low as 18, 37 or 42 nmol. These levels are very low and it is very hard for you to have healthy skin with such low levels. In fact, one young Indian male was very distressed because he had acne on his arms, legs, face, back and chest. His result was 16 nmol, one of the lowest I have seen. Once we returned his vitamin D level to normal his acne disappeared. Darker skin types as well as people who suffer dry skin will not absorb and make vitamin D in the same way as lighter skinned people. This means if this is you that you need to be more vigilant in checking your vitamin D annually and if you have a skin condition it should be one of the first things you do to start on the road to health.*

Due to the fact that skin conditions and vitamin D deficiency go hand in hand, I would strongly recommend that you have your vitamin D levels checked. In Australia and New Zealand they need to be around 75 nmol and above. I like to see my clients over 100 nmol to support healing and healthy hormonal function.

For countries such as the USA, Ginde[11,13], in a nutritional article published in *Scientific America*, linked vitamin D deficiency to catching more colds, blaming the increasing use of sunscreen and long sleeves following skin cancer and prevention campaigns for the change. Using a sunscreen with as little as a 15-factor protection cuts the skin's vitamin D production by 99%, the study noted, and there are few sources of the vitamin in our diets. Some food sources are salmon, tuna, mackerel and vitamin D-fortified dairy products, such as milk — which is over-processed and pasteurised, leaving very little vitamin D available for absorption.

Depending on the colour of your skin, darker skinned people should take double the amount of vitamin D supplements, because they have more melanin or pigment in their skin that makes it harder for their body to absorb and use the sun's ultraviolet rays to synthesise vitamin D. It is also important in winter to increase your vitamin D when there is less sun exposure.

Facts about water

Water is one of the most vital elements to enable us to sustain life. Making up about 65–70% of our body, it is no wonder it is vital for our cells as it supports cellular hydration, regulates the temperature of our body, carries nutrients to our cells and flushes out cellular waste, allowing toxins to be removed.

If our body and skin cells are starved of water, they become shrivelled-up, parched and dry, making it easy for viruses and diseases to attack. It is important to drink not only sufficient water every day but also clean, healthy, toxin- and fluoride-free water, together with consuming fresh vegetables and fruit that have not been commercially prepared and put in long life packets.

Illness and degeneration of your health can result from long consumption of unhealthy, toxic water and unhealthy foods and failing to exercise! If you are like most people you will be more inclined to drink when you are thirsty rather than for health. It is for this reason that it is important to keep track of your fluid intake when you start to change this habit to make sure you meet your quota rather than drinking reactively. Your skin uses water in the form of sweat as a process of detoxification and so constantly supporting this process, especially after exercise, is vital to good skin health.

It is estimated that without exercise included, the average adult loses 6.3 cups of water a day through urination and an additional 4 cups through other bodily functions such as bowel movements, perspiration and breathing.[35] To make up this deficit, it is recommended to drink 8–9 cups of water per day or approximately 1–2 litres. Of course, if you are exercising for an hour you should add another 1.5–2.5 cups and if you are living in a warmer climate or at higher altitudes you will require more again on top of the 8–9 cups.

It is important that you don't include or count sugary drinks such as cola, cordial, coffee and tea in your daily intake as these are separate and counterproductive to good hydration. In fact, they increase water loss because they act as a diuretic — which means they make you urinate more — so you need to add an extra cup of water for every cup of coffee, tea, and sugary drinks that you consume.

Also, remember that it is not advised to include sugary drinks in a healthy skin and body programme. They create so many problems with your body's sugar balance and hormonal health that it is best to completely avoid them.

As you can see, adequate clean water is essential for skin, body and mental health. In fact, inadequate water intake can lead to mild or moderate dehydration with significant symptoms that you may not have considered previously. These symptoms are:

- Acne
- Bloating
- Confusion
- Constipation
- Cramps in arms or legs
- Urine that is dark in colour
- Decreased urine output
- Digestive problems, including heartburn and stomach ache
- Dizziness
- Dry eyes and skin
- Dry mouth
- Extreme thirst
- Fatigue
- Flushed face
- Headaches

- Irritability
- Loss of appetite
- Low back pain
- Low blood pressure
- Nosebleeds
- Poor concentration
- Recurring urinary tract infections
- Sinus problems
- Soreness of muscles and joints
- Water retention

Electricity travels over water, and nerve impulses also travel via water; therefore, without water your body cannot control and regulate its nervous system correctly, leaving you with less than optimal health, skin dehydration and reduced healing capacity and wellbeing.

If you don't have a water filter, I would suggest that you consider installing one or buy yourself a container such as a jug or water bottle that includes one. Make a point of filtering your water and ensure that you change the filter regularly. In Australia our tap water can contain traces of pollutants such as:

- **Pesticides** — Levels are regulated, but the Australian limit for Lindane, for instance, is 200 times the allowable European limit. Toxic effects include: cancer, multiple sclerosis, Parkinson's disease, and male Infertility and hormonal imbalance.
- **Chloroform** — A by-product of chlorine, which can cause reproductive problems, brain damage and can be toxic to the skin and lungs.
- **PCBs** — Added to plastics and used in some domestic piping.
- **Benzene** — Absorbed at small but significant levels from atmospheric pollution can cause drowsiness, dizziness, headaches, confusion, rapid heart rate, unconsciousness, coma and even death. Benzene can also affect the reproductive organs and can cause low birthweights, delayed bone formation and bone marrow damage in unborn foetuses.

- **Mercury** — Symptoms of exposure are: fatigue, memory loss, mental disorders and headaches. Toxic effects include: heart attack, angina, deafness, kidney damage, Hodgkin's disease, liver damage, arthritis, muscle tension and weakness, Alzheimer's disease and autism. Mercury can also cause Infertility in both sexes and birth defects.
- **Lead** — Can easily be absorbed from old plumbing, soldering joints and tanks. Toxic effects include: anaemia, high blood pressure, colic, constipation, deafness, kidney damage, cancer, liver damage, brain damage, dementia, insomnia, male infertility and miscarriages.
- **Bacteria** and other organisms like *Giardia* and so on. Symptoms of exposure are: diarrhoea, bloating, belching, gut pain, ulcers, dysentery and lung disease.
- **Chemicals** — Many of the pollutants added by man include fluoride. Fluoride can cause mottled teeth, reduce thyroid function below optimum, cause bone disorders such as osteoporosis, hyperactivity, weak muscles, gastric pains, vomiting and nausea, irritable bowel syndrome, headaches, vertigo, spasticity, and has been linked to cancer, heart disease, diabetes and cot death.
- **Raw sewage**.
- **Industrial waste**.

As well as all of these, practically all municipal drinking water contains the inorganic mineral calcium carbonate. Calcium carbonate, and other inorganic minerals, can cause all kinds of stones to form in our vital organs, cement our joints and is the principal troublemaker responsible for what is called "hardening of the arteries", that is solidifying our blood vessels. Calcium carbonate, or lime, is a very important ingredient in making cement or concrete, and we all know that adding water to cement leads to hardening of concrete. The most common places to find the accumulation of such stones are in the gall bladder, the kidneys, and in the passageways between the kidneys and the bladder.

Calcium carbonate is something we can definitely do without and the best way to eliminate this substance, heavy metals and the above list of toxins is to buy a water filter. There are several types from a simple carbon filter, to reverse osmosis, distillation and alkalising filters.

So make sure that the water you are drinking is good quality and supports your goals of health, vitality and glowing skin. Do your research and avoid plastic bottles and containers, unless they carry the triangle sign with a number two or above inside it. This means that is hardened plastic and not likely to leach any of its components when exposed to extreme heat, (such as a water bottle sitting in your car during summer), or cold.

Dairy and its effect on skin

It is often hard to know what foods to eat, how to prepare them and how to get the best from what you eat. We are marketed to so heavily around food that it is hard to know where the truth lies. I hope that this section about dairy will help you sift the wheat from the chaff by firstly taking you back to basics.

Let's start with dairy and milk products. The typical Western diet includes the consumption of a lot of milk. In the UK alone, consumers buy around 5.2 billion litres of liquid milk from the supermarkets and the milkman each year. On top of that, 6 billion litres go into dairy products such as cheese, butter and dried milk powder, which is a vital component of many other food products. All in all, we buy enough dairy products every year to fill nearly 4,500 Olympic-size swimming pools![36]

So, my question is, do we rely too much on milk for our nutritional (calcium) support?

Firstly, we get more calcium from our greens than we do from dairy — I mean, ask yourself, where do you think the cows get their calcium from?

Lactose is a disaccharide or milk sugar and if we are to eat/digest milk we need to make this enzyme. The enzyme needed to break down any dairy product is called β-galactosidase or lactase and it is normally present only during infancy and childhood; therefore allowing the young to acquire energy from their mother's milk and growth factor.

Knowing that lactose is a sugar, if you are on any health/weight loss programme you may want to rethink consumption of dairy products as all dairy turns to fat if it is not used as energy. This simply means that sugar is converted into fat for storage when it is not used in your daily energy expenditure.

Historically, our European descendants, due to genetic predisposition or adaption, where there was an abundance of plant food/greens available all year round, did not include a high content of milk products in their diet. It was only in the colder climates where snow fell and there were fewer greens to support health that cows' and goats' milk was introduced and adapted into the diet and has remained there today.

Symptoms such as rectal gas, feelings of indigestion, acne and bloating may be signs that you are not producing lactase.

In our Westernised, dairy-based diet, dairy products have now been pasteurised, sanitised and homogenised to the point where there is very little nutritional value left and, unfortunately, what you are left with is the chemical skeleton of what milk used to be and therefore an increase in allergens.

According to natural health experts Dr Cordain, Dr Mercola and Dr Wartian Smith[3,1,9,21,36,] you may think differently about the next time you have milk products because they say:

"The path that transforms healthy milk products into allergens and carcinogens begins with modern feeding methods that substitute high-protein, soy-based feeds for fresh green grass and breeding methods to produce cows with abnormally large pituitary glands so that they produce three times more milk than the old fashioned scrub cow."

Dairy and its connection to skin disorders has been well researched and documented, especially in relation to acne.[36] The main causal factor, other than the manipulation of the milk itself, is the fact that there is an abundance of a hormone called IGF-1 in milk, which is okay for baby cows because that is who it has been produced for, not for you/us as humans. IGF-1 is a growth hormone. It makes calves grow into cows, but in humans, it tends to make your acne grow big instead as it overstimulates the sebaceous gland in your skin to produce more oil. IGF-1 is one of several factors that cause inflammation in humans, and which eventually leads to acne (and the ugly redness and swelling that makes acne so annoying).

Milk and dairy products also cause an insulin spike in humans that causes the liver to produce even more IGF-1, leading to even more acne. This means you get locked into a vicious cycle when you eat dairy. The best way to avoid this is to eliminate butter, cream, cheese, yoghurt and milk! *(Note: an exception to this rule is kefir yoghurt.)*

In summary, I have listed below the effects that dairy products have on your skin:

- Dairy causes your skin to produce excess sebum (oil), leading to — you guessed it! — more clogged pores, more acne, and a breeding ground for *Propionibacterium acnes*, which feed on your sebum and spew out inflammatory by-products.
- Dairy glues together dead skin cells inside your pores, so they can't exit naturally, leading to clogged pores (and thus more acne).

My recommendation to clients and to you is to eliminate milk and dairy products from your diet and add greens and almonds if you are worried about your calcium levels. Use nut milks instead of dairy and check your iodine levels and hormonal levels to keep your bones healthy and strong and you will be happier, healthier and leaner.

Dairy alternatives: a quick glance

Table 9: Dairy alternatives

Food	Suggested Alternatives
Milk	Nut milks such as almond, cashew
	Soy milk if not low thyroid, iodine or high oestrogen
	Oat milk — check brands for excess sugar added
Butter	Ghee
	Dairy-free margarine
	Avocado spread
	Coconut oil
Cheese	There are some great vegan cheeses available. I like the ones made with almond butter or coconut oil, for example Vegusto
	Soy cheese, if not high in oestrogen or low in iodine or thyroid function
Yoghurt	Kefir — has amazing anti-yeast, probiotic benefits
	There are also coconut-based yoghurts available now in Australia
Cream	I have a great recipe for cashew cream that goes great with any dessert plus add a little vinegar and you have sour cream!
Ice cream	There are a variety of ice creams that use bases such as cashews and coconut, so if you are after a sweet treat, check them out at your local health food shop or gourmet deli. But, remember to check the amount of sugar and choose stevia and xylitol sweeteners over raw sugar and sucrose.

Food allergies

Have you ever experienced watery eyes, nasal congestion, bloating after meals, diarrhoea or found yourself sniffling and sneezing after meals? You may have some food allergies or intolerances that are contributing to or creating your skin condition.

Food allergies can cause these symptoms as well as make you crave the food you're allergic too! Sounds crazy doesn't it! However, if you consider the additives, colourings and preservatives that are added to our food and the way they are manufactured, it is no surprise that our bodies and skin may well be suffering as these inorganic compounds find their way into our bodies day after day after day.

So, what is a food allergy?

A food allergy occurs when your body shows a hypersensitivity to a normally harmless substance in our environment. When you come into contact with this substance, also called an allergen, it triggers your body's immune response to release a substance called histamine. These histamines widen your blood vessels, causing inflammation, which allows protein called antibodies to get to the tissue affected and neutralise the allergen. While an allergic reaction can be caused through airborne substances such as dust and pollen, the most common food allergens are dairy products (butter, cream, cheese, milk), eggs, peanuts, tree nuts such as almonds, cashews and walnuts, seafood, soy, wheat, and so on.

Sometimes a negative food reaction may be a food intolerance rather than an allergy.[34] In this case, the problem is that the body does not have/make the necessary enzymes to break down the food properly and often dietary enzymes can help with this. However, it is my experience that eliminating the main allergens, dairy and wheat, is the best place to start and monitor your reactions once this has been done. I would also recommend that you have your iodine levels checked as iodine supports the healthy production of stomach acid (called hydrochloric acid), and acts as a stomach antiseptic, therefore protecting you from harmful foods, bacteria and so on.

The amount of food necessary to cause a reaction in a person differs, as does the severity of the symptoms that range from mild to life-threatening. Generally, a food allergy will result in one or more of the physical symptoms:

- Abdominal pain
- Acne
- Anal itching
- Anaphylaxis
- Anaemia
- Backache
- Breathing difficulties
- Canker sores
- Chest pain
- Cracks at the corners of the mouth
- Dark circles under the eyes
- Diarrhoea
- Dizziness
- Eczema
- Fatigue
- Fluid retention
- Food cravings
- Frequent urination
- Gas
- Headaches
- Heartburn
- Hives
- Hoarseness
- Itchy, watery eyes
- Itchy skin
- Low blood pressure
- Muscle aches
- Nasal congestion

- Nausea
- Persistent cough
- Rash or hives
- Reddened earlobes, eyes or cheeks
- Ringing in the ears
- Stomach cramps
- Tension headaches
- Tremors
- Wrinkles under the eyes

Research has also shown that there is a link between allergies and a number of mental and emotional symptoms such as[49]:

- Anxiety
- Attention deficit disorder
- Brain fog
- Compulsive behaviour
- Disorientation dyslexia
- Emotional outbursts
- Epilepsy
- Irritability
- Lethargy
- Memory loss
- Mood swings
- Panic attacks
- Paranoia
- Restlessness
- Weepiness

Whilst food intolerances share many of the same symptoms as food allergies, the majority of the complaints centre on your digestive tract. Therefore, you may be suffering an intolerance if you are experiencing one or more of the symptoms below after eating:

- Diarrhoea
- Gas, cramps or bloating
- Headaches
- Heartburn
- Irritability or nervousness
- Nausea
- Stomach pains
- Vomiting

Food allergies and intolerances are a complex issue, so it is best to get the advice of a natural health practitioner to help you. However, it is always helpful to keep a diary to monitor your symptoms, if any, after eating and note any patterns.

Clinical note:

All my clients tell me about their experience with acne breakout within 48 hours of ingesting dairy. In fact, it is usually within 24 hours. Clients suffering from rosacea do not describe such obvious change, some clients have reported that their flare-ups and flushing is generally worse after eating dairy and any foods with high sugar content.

Understand your sugar cravings

For many years, scientists and nutritionists have preached that weight loss comes down to a simple equation: kilojoules in versus kilojoules out. While this principle is true to an extent, there are a number of increasingly common *hormonal shifts* that can alter this relationship. Insulin resistance[8,25,34,] the clinical condition that precedes type 2 diabetes, is one such condition. Individuals with insulin resistance will struggle to lose weight via traditional weight loss prescriptions simply because their body is not burning fuel the way it should be.

Insulin is a hormone secreted by the pancreas that is used to digest carbohydrates. Carbohydrates are found in plant-based foods, including bread, rice, breakfast cereal, pasta, fruits and sugars. When carbohydrate-rich foods are consumed, insulin is secreted by the pancreas to take glucose from the food to the muscles to produce energy. For a number of reasons, over time insulin may fail to work as well as it should. Weight gain, where fat clogs the cells, is one reason, *as is a lack of physical activity.* Genes can also predispose a person to insulin resistance and type 2 diabetes.

The highly processed nature of our daily carbohydrate food choices, including breads, breakfast cereals and snack foods, which require much higher amounts of insulin than less processed, low-GI carbohydrates, is also thought to be a significant contributing factor to the increased incidence of insulin resistance. Resistance to insulin builds up over time, with the body gradually demanding but not necessarily producing more insulin in an attempt to support optimum health and energy.

As insulin is also a fat-storing hormone, the more of it that circulates in the body, the harder it becomes to burn body fat. High levels of insulin can also make you feel tired, bloated and crave sugar: a bit like food intolerance, wouldn't you say? Individuals with insulin resistance also tend to have distinct abdominal fat deposits, and carry much of their weight around their belly. However, once diagnosed, managing insulin resistance can prevent the development of type 2 diabetes. While some cases may warrant medication, I would suggest that before you start medication you have your thyroid health: T4, T3 and iodine levels checked first, as these alone need to be addressed to manage insulin resistance. Then if you do need medication you will get the best results; however, in my experience this is not often until the thyroid and the iodine levels are returned to normal.

So why are we talking about insulin resistance when this is a book on skin health and wellness? Well, it may come as no surprise to you that untamed insulin levels will also affect your skin with the resultant conditions being types 1 and 2 acne, and contributing to types 1, 2 and 3 rosacea. So, if you have these conditions *(see "Insulin resistance questionnaire" on page 100)*. I would suggest that you overhaul your diet even more to reduce the effects of your food choices/refined carbohydrates that are affecting your skin's health.

Individuals with insulin resistance need to reduce carbohydrates, increase protein foods such as chicken, fish, eggs and meat, as well as integrating a training programme of moderate-intensity cardiovascular sessions with a light resistance training programme. Interval training is one of the best ways to start reducing insulin resistance as well as making sure that you increase your incidental activity and walk a minimum of 10,000 steps or approximately 7.5 kilometres a day. Individuals with insulin resistance need to become fussy with their choice of carbohydrates. High-GI, refined sources of carbohydrates, including fruit juice, white bread and refined cereals and pastas should be completely eliminated from your diet if you are serious.

To explain a little more about how sugar has increased its effect on us, let me give you a snapshot of the history of sugar and how it affects our body so you can understand what's happening in your body a little better. This, in turn, I hope, will help you make the decisions to implement changes.

Sugar, sweeteners and their history

Sugar cane is one of the oldest cultivated crops known to man. In fact, sugar and honey are the oldest natural sweeteners.

Sugar has been globally traded throughout the centuries as a valuable commodity. As early as 6000 BC, there are indications of primitive sugar production from sugar cane in New Guinea, where the people were chewing and sucking the stalks of the sweet juice. Sugar cane cultivation spread to India, where by 500 BC people had learned to turn bowls of juice from the tropical grass into crude crystals. From there, sugar travelled with migrants and monks to China, Persia, Northern Africa and eventually to Europe in the 11th century.

You might ask why sugar is so popular or why is it such a valuable commodity. Well, considering that every single cell in our body depends on sugar for energy and your brain is the largest user, you can understand how your body has developed this desire, dependence and demand for sweet tastes and our problem is we feed it!

The amount of sugar we consume has changed dramatically over time, as it has with many foods and manufacturing methods. Before agriculture, our ancestors presumably did not have much control over the sugars in their diet, which must have come from whatever plants and animals were available in a given geographical area and season.

Sugar — brown or white and high fructose corn syrup — their effects on your body

Today, we add sugar in one form or another to the majority of processed foods we eat — everything from bread, cereals, processed foods, desserts, soft drinks, juices, salad dressings and sauces — and we are not too stingy about using it to sweeten many raw and wholefoods as well.

In the early 1980s, high-fructose corn syrup (HFCS) replaced sugar in carbonated soft drinks and other products, in part because refined sugar then had the reputation as a generally noxious nutrient. ("Villain in Disguise?" asked a headline in 1977, before answering in the affirmative.[6]) HFCS was portrayed by the food industry as a healthy alternative and that's how the public perceived it. It was also cheaper than sugar, which didn't hurt its commercial prospects. Now the tide is turning the other way, and refined sugar is making a commercial comeback as the supposedly healthy alternative to this noxious HFCS. Industry after industry is replacing their product with sucrose and advertising it as such, with the words "No High-Fructose Corn Syrup".[7] Gary Taubes and Loren Cordain noted, when completing their research into the addition of HFCS in our diets, that not only was there an increase in heart disease, stress disorders and diabetes, but young girls were beginning puberty as young as eight years old, rather than the acceptable 16 years old and this could be directly linked back to the increase in the use of HFCS in your processed packaged foods and snacks.[6]

By consuming large quantities of sugar, we are not just demonstrating weak willpower and indulging our sweet tooth — we are, in fact, poisoning ourselves according to a group of doctors, nutritionists and biologists. One of the most prominent members of this group is Robert Lustig, of the University of California, San Francisco, famous for his viral YouTube video *Sugar: The Bitter Truth*. A few journalists, such as Gary Taubes and Mark Bittman, have reached similar conclusions.[6,7,8,10] Sugar, they argue, poses far greater dangers than cavities and love handles; it is a toxin that harms our organs and disrupts the body's usual hormonal cycles. For skin conditions this spells disaster and as the hormonal disruption affects the health of your skin in the form of acne, rosacea and persistent redness as well as skin tags and excess skin growths.

Sugar or fructose: which one is the hormonal disruptor?

More than 6 million Australian adults and approximately 6 million children and adolescents in Australia are overweight or obese.

The human body strictly regulates the amount of glucose in the blood. Glucose stimulates the pancreas to secrete the hormone insulin, as previously discussed, which helps remove excess glucose from blood, and bolsters production of the hormone leptin, which suppresses hunger. Fructose, which is twice as sweet as sucrose, does not trigger insulin production and appears to raise levels of the hormone grehlin, which keeps us hungry. Some researchers have suggested that large amounts of fructose encourage people to eat more than they need due to this fact.[7]

On average, people in Australia, America and Europe eat between 100 and 150 grams of sugar each day, about half of which is fructose. It's difficult to find a regional diet or individual food that contains only glucose or only fructose. Virtually all plants have glucose, fructose and sucrose — not just one of these sugars. Although some fruits, such as apples and pears, have three times as much fructose as glucose, most of the fruits and vegetables we eat are more balanced. Pineapples, blueberries, peaches, carrots, corn and cabbage, for example, all have about a 1:1 ratio of the two sugars.

Super-sugary, energy-dense foods, with little nutritional value, are one of the main ways we consume more calories than we need, albeit not the only way. It might be hard to swallow, but the fact is that many of your favourite desserts, snacks, cereals and especially your beloved sweet beverages inundate the body with far more sugar than it is able to efficiently metabolise. This, in turn, directs and overstimulates your body's digestive hormone insulin and your stress hormones are activated to bring our sugar levels back into balance, which, together with insulin, create a balance similar to the action a thermostat-programmed to keep a room at a constant 25° Celsius.[1] The problems arise again not long after the sugar has been metabolised and within 30 minutes the blood sugar levels plummet and your stress hormones adrenaline and cortisol are needed again to rebalance your blood sugar levels to keep you clear-headed and upright. The milkshakes, smoothies, carbonated drinks, energy drinks and even unsweetened fruit juices all contain large amounts of free-floating sugars instantly absorbed by our digestive system, sending your blood sugar levels into a swing of highs and lows.

So how does this affect your skin?

As the body goes through the swings of highs and lows from food intake, the microcirculation in the skin is affected by this hormonal response. When the body is stressed, the microcirculation in the skin responds to the hormonal stress stimulus by reducing capillaries' blood flow and encourages more blood flow into the deeper tissues and organs to support digestion, metabolism and normalisation.[1] This is a problem for the skin as fewer nutrients and less oxygen are available to optimise its health.

The sebaceous gland, another structure in the skin, is influenced by this stress as well as the reduction in microcirculation and, to compensate, under or over secretes oily sebum, which results in either excess sebum on the skin's surface and oily skin with dehydration, or dry skin with dehydration again. In conditions such as acne and rosacea, these swings in blood sugar encourage harmful bacterial overgrowth and destabilise the pH balance of the skin, making it difficult for the skin to stay in balance, again resulting in increased stress within the microcirculation, redness, congestion and sensitivity.

Last, but not least, is the premature ageing that occurs when the blood sugars in the body are constantly swinging from big highs to big lows over a period of years. These affects can be seen on the skin in the form of skin tags that occur around the neck, armpits and chest as a result of prolonged and chronic congestion and a decrease in oxygenation to the skin.

Oh gosh! What do I need to do?

Avoiding sugar is not an answer on its own as there are natural sugars in fruits and vegetables. A better approach is to reduce the processed sugar that you put in your cup of tea/coffee and keeping the cookies out of reach or hidden in the cupboard. Then there's all the stuff we really should eat more of: whole grains; fruits and vegetables; fish; and lean protein. But wait, you can't stop there: a balanced diet is only one component of a healthy lifestyle. We need to exercise too — to get our hearts pumping, strengthen our muscles and bones, use the energy we have available and maintain flexibility. Taubes states:

> *"Exercising, favouring wholefoods over-processed ones and eating less overall sounds too obvious, too simplistic, but it is actually a far more nuanced approach to good health than vilifying a single molecule in our diet.*[7]*"*

In the Western world we have continued to consume more and more total calories each year — our average daily intake increased by 530 calories between 1970 and 2010 — while simultaneously becoming less and less physically active and dealing with lives that are getting busier and busier. Here's the bitter truth: yes, most of us should make an effort to eat less sugar — but if we are really committed to staying healthy and improving the health of our skin, we'll have to do a lot more than that as the years roll on.

If you think that you may be insulin resistant or wondering if sugar is affecting your health and your skin, then complete the questionnaire. If you are positive to insulin resistance, the recipes and food programme at the end of this section are a great resource to help you get back on track until you feel more confident with experimenting for yourself.

Insulin resistance questionnaire

Do you carry most of your extra weight around your abdominal area?

☐ No

☐ A little

☐ Yes, most of my excess weight sits around my stomach area

Do you tend to put on weight easily?

☐ No

☐ Yes, if I eat more than usual

☐ Yes, even without excessive overeating

Do you battle to lose weight when following a diet?

☐ No or never follow a diet or not overweight

☐ Depends on the diet

☐ Never normally have success losing weight

Is there a family history of or do you suffer from any of the following: diabetes, heart disease such as high cholesterol or high blood pressure or gout?

☐ No

☐ Yes, at least one of these apply to me or my family

☐ Yes, more than one of these apply to me or my family

If female, do you have polycystic ovarian syndrome?

☐ No, not that I am aware, or not female

☐ Yes

Do you suffer with fluid retention in general?

☐ No

☐ At certain times of the month for example, premenstrual

☐ Often

If female, do you suffer from premenstrual tension including food cravings and mood swings?

☐ No, or I am a male

☐ Some months

☐ Every month

Do you suffer from depression?

☐ No

☐ Unsure

☐ Yes

Do you experience frequent food cravings, especially for sugary or starchy foods?

☐ No

☐ Yes

☐ All the time

Do your food cravings, especially for sweet or starchy foods, occur later in the day, especially late afternoon and evening?

☐ No, or no cravings

☐ Sometimes

☐ Most of the time

Do you suffer from mood swings?

☐ No

☐ Sometimes

☐ All the time

Are you usually tired or suffer from fatigue in the afternoon or early evening?

☐ So

☐ Sometimes

☐ Most days

Have you experienced any of the following: unexplained weight loss, excessive thirst, frequent urination?

☐ No

☐ Yes, at least one of the above

☐ At least two of the above

Do you find it hard to maintain your mental focus, especially in the afternoon?

☐ Yes

☐ No

☐ Sometimes

Now add up your score. If you said yes to two or more of these questions, you should be eliminating all processed sugars and carbohydrates and making sure you are exercising for at least 30 minutes a day. Check out the food planner and recipes at the end of Section Two and start enjoying balance!

The food programme at the end of Section Two is designed to help you get started on a healthier eating plan and give you some recipes to start moving towards healthier choices. It has not been designed as a weight loss programme; however, if you are making better, healthier choices you may find that you do lose some weight as your body stabilises your hormones and digestion and you sleep more soundly.

If you have type 2 acne or have been diagnosed with polycystic ovary disease (PCOS), I would suggest that you remove all fruit for at least one month and commence a probiotic such with the beneficial strain saccharomyces boulardii. Once your skin has cleared, you may add one serving of fruit such as an apple a day, but not concentrated fruit juice on its own.

Enjoy!

SLEEP

૭

The importance of a good night's sleep can never be understated. The difference that an extra hour of sleep on a regular, nightly basis makes in your life may be quite a lot, experts say.[4] Studies show that the gap between getting just enough sleep and getting too little sleep may affect your health, your mood, your weight, and even your sex life. Make a point of starting your bed routine at about 9.30 pm so you are in bed with lights out by 10.00 pm. A cool room with good ventilation and effective block out is also important for a good night of uninterrupted sleep as your body needs to reduce its temperature to go to sleep and stay asleep.

If you're getting less than the recommended eight hours of sleep a night I want to give you nine good reasons to shut down your computer, television or electronic device, turn off the lights and hit the bed for some shut-eye.[4, 22]

- **Healthy glowing skin and low blood glucose.** When it comes to being a supermodel they always make sure that they prepare for their shoot by sleeping at least eight hours a night. Not sleeping enough can lead to unhealthy and unattractive skin (fine lines, wrinkles, acne, lacklustre skin, and so on).

- **Better sex life**. According to a poll conducted by the National Sleep Foundation, up to 26% of people say that their sex lives tend to suffer because they're just too tired. There's evidence that in men, impaired sleep can be associated with lower testosterone levels — although the exact nature of the link isn't clear.

- **Less pain.** If you have chronic pain — or acute pain from a recent injury — getting enough sleep may actually make you hurt less. Many studies have shown a link between sleep loss and a lower pain threshold. Unfortunately, being in pain can make it hard to sleep. *(Check out the information on grounding/ earthing on page 106 — I have found this invaluable for aches, pains and general inflammation.)*

- **Lower risk of injury.** Sleeping enough might actually keep you safer. Sleep deprivation has been linked with many road vehicle accidents. The Institute of Medicine estimates that one out of five automobile accidents in the USA alone results from drowsy driving — that's about one million crashes a year. We in Australia follow a similar pattern. Of course, when you're overtired you're also more likely to trip, fall off a ladder, or cut yourself while chopping vegetables due to lack of attention.

- **Better mood.** Getting enough sleep won't guarantee a sunny disposition. But you have probably noticed that when you're exhausted, you're more likely to be cranky. That's not all. Not getting enough sleep affects your emotional regulators and when you're overtired, you're more likely to snap at your boss, burst into tears or start laughing uncontrollably.

- **Better weight control.** Getting enough sleep could help you maintain your weight — and, conversely, sleep loss goes with an increased risk of weight gain. Why? Part of the problem is behavioural. If you're overtired, you might be less likely to have the energy to go for that jog or cook a healthy dinner after work. The other part is physiological. The hormone Leptin plays a key role in making you feel full. ***When you don't get enough sleep***, Leptin levels drop. The bottom line is people who are tired are just plain hungrier and they seem to crave high-fat and high-calorie foods, specifically because they are after the energy boost.

- **Clearer thinking.** Have you ever woken up after a bad night's sleep, feeling fuzzy and easily confused, like your brain can't get out of first gear? "Sleep loss affects how you think. It impairs your cognition, your attention, and your decision-making.[4]" Studies have found that people who are sleep-deprived are substantially worse at solving logic, and have reduced mental clarity for problem solving and mathematical problems than when they're well rested.

- **Better memory.** Feeling forgetful? Sleep loss could be to blame. Studies have shown that while we sleep, our brains process and consolidate our memories from the day. If you don't get enough sleep, those memories might not get stored correctly and can be lost.
- **Stronger immunity.** Could getting enough sleep prevent the common cold? One preliminary study put the idea to the test. Researchers tracked over 150 people and monitored their sleep habits for two weeks. Then they exposed them to a cold virus. People who got seven hours of sleep a night or less were almost three times as likely to get sick as the people who got at least eight hours of sleep a night.

How do you know if you are getting enough sleep?

Your sleep is affected by the everyday stresses you experience every day. This stress affects your blood glucose levels, energy, mental clarity, digestive microbiome and your body's ability to repair itself. Excess stress and poor sleep will encourage premature ageing and inflammation, reflecting in an imbalance in your body as well as your skin.

This imbalance can certainly show in the form of acne, rosacea, eczema, psoriasis and skin rashes. Therefore, your skin condition could well be a symptom of this long-term imbalance or your lack of sleep may well be a contributing factor to slow healing and regular flare-ups. So, make sure you get to bed by 10 pm and have a restful eight hours of sleep. If you are getting good-quality sleep you should wake refreshed, clear-headed and ready for the day.

If you are not feeling like this then you may want to do the oestrogen dominance questionnaire *(on page 54)* and go through the chapter "Your skin and your hormonal health: the complex connection" *(on page 30)* to review how your stress and metabolic hormones affect your skin and health.

Our skin and body connection with sleep

What ages our bodies and our skin, whether or not we have a skin condition, is inflammation!

As we discussed previously, your skin condition may well be a symptom rather than a condition. When the skin and body are inflamed and out of balance, you will have an active immune system that is producing free radicals to try and reduce the inflammation and bring the body back into balance.

Another way of reducing inflammation and promoting a good night's sleep is by grounding yourself while you sleep. Your connection to nature, the planet and the universe is a fundamental part of your existence as a human being. However, with rapid advances in technology, changes to architecture, your modern, fast-paced lifestyles, changes in your food chain, including changes in farming methods that include the integration of herbicides as well as pesticides, chemically loaded personal care products usage as well as home care, preparation and packaging of food, many of us have become separated from our basic bond with Mother Earth. When was the last time you walked barefoot on the earth, or anywhere for that matter? We are so busy and time-poor that we drive to most places, already thinking about the next task. I know that I have been guilty of that!

We all know that the sun gives us warmth, life, light and vitamin D and the earth provides us with fresh air, water, food, and a surface to live on. However, it has recently been discovered that when your bare feet make contact with the earth's surface, your body takes up a natural and subtle energy in the form of electrons that have a negative charge — we call this vitamin G. This could be the difference between feeling good and not so good, or having little or a lot of energy, sleeping well or not so well, looking vibrant or looking tired and old.

Throughout history, humans walked barefoot, slept on the ground, cultivated their land with bare hands and spent a lot of their time naturally grounded. However, we have become increasingly disconnected from nature by our modern lifestyle. The conductive, leather-soled shoes of our ancestors have been replaced with insulated rubber and plastics that were introduced in the 1960s. We sleep in beds and homes off the ground. Your home and office surround you with electronic devices, wireless connections, microwaves and cell towers, which assault us continuously with a positive charge.

The earth's surface is negatively charged, full of free electrons, ready and waiting for us. As human beings living in today's world, every single one of us is bursting full of destructive, positively charged free radicals that cause inflammation and damage to our bodies. Many of us have become electron-deficient and lopsided with a positive charge. This positive charge results in subtle, yet accumulative damage and increased inflammation to your body's cells, including your skin.

When you connect to the earth with your bare skin your body becomes infused with negatively charged electrons, which means you neutralise the excess, positively charged free radicals, which prevent damage to healthy tissue and normalise your immune response, thus returning your body to normal when healing can occur. Research shows that at least 45 minutes a day is what is needed to start making positive changes to your body and skin.[33]

Revolutionary new research by Clint Ober has raised the possibility that this disconnection and lack of electrons may actually contribute to chronic pain, fatigue, poor sleep and autoimmune diseases that plague so many of us today.[33]

The remedy for this modern-day disconnect is simple. Walk barefoot outdoors whenever possible and/or sleep, work, or relax indoors in contact with conductive sheets or mats that transfer the energy to your body in the comfort of your home or office when it suits you. People who do this on a regular basis say they sleep better, feel better, have more energy during the day and look better. This simple practice is both a technology and a movement, which is transforming lives across the planet and is known as "earthing".

Earthing is safe and natural, for people of all ages, young and old, but it is not medicine or a substitute for medical treatment if you are acutely ill.

How can I experience earthing now?

Go barefoot outside for at least half an hour to 45 minutes and see what a difference it makes to your pain or stress level.[31-33] Sit, stand or walk on grass, sand, dirt, or plain concrete. These are all conductive surfaces from which your body can draw the earth's energy. Wood, asphalt, sealed or painted concrete and vinyl won't work. They are not conductive surfaces. Other ways to earth yourself:

- Swim in the ocean or lakes.
- Garden with bare hands.
- Lie on the earth.
- Hug a tree.
- Sleep on the earth while camping.
- Wear natural, leather-soled shoes instead of synthetic rubber/plastic shoes.
- Wear conductive-soled shoes.
- Use indoor conductive earthing products such as sheets and mats.

Earthing is a great and easy way to improve your skin's health as it helps restore your body's balance reduces inflammation and promotes healing as well as skin cell renewal without you lifting a finger.

Apart from assisting the improvement of your skin's health and healing, earthing or grounding is reported to assist with other body imbalances such as:

- Improve or eliminate the symptoms of many inflammation-related disorders.
- Reduce or eliminate chronic pain.
- Improve sleep — resulting in deeper, more refreshing sleep.
- Increase energy levels.
- Lower stress and promote calmness in the body by cooling down the nervous system and stress hormones.
- Normalise the body's biological rhythms and cortisol levels.
- Thinning the blood and improve blood pressure and flow.

- Relieve muscle tension and headaches.
- Lessen hormonal and menstrual symptoms.
- Dramatically speed healing and help prevent bedsores.
- Reduce or eliminate jet lag.
- Protect the body against potentially health-disturbing environmental electromagnetic fields (EMFs).
- Accelerate recovery from intense athletic activity (for example, earthing sheets were used by the Tour de France athletes to aid recovery from the day's riding with a great outcome for the riders).

I love the benefits of earthing and it's just another healthy body support that keeps me healthy, supports vitality and reduces skin ageing. The best thing about earthing is that you can do it while you sleep if you have an earthing sheet so there is no effort! One final comment about earthing is if you decide to get the sheets for your bed and enjoy the benefits of grounding while you sleep the secret to successful grounding comes from sleeping *au naturale*. The more your skin is in contact with the sheet the more grounded you are.

Clinical note:

When I first experienced grounding I noticed straight away that my skin experienced some tingling. That seemed to fade after about half an hour and I noticed that I certainly slept well that night. But what impressed on me the value of the grounding sheets the most was the experience that I had when I came back from a business trip. I didn't sleep very well at the hotel and after two days I was really looking forward to being in my own bed. The first night home was the best night's sleep I had had in three days. It really demonstrated to me the contrast between being grounded versus sleeping on a normal sheet. It was such a difference that I bought a sheet to take away with me whenever I travel now.

STRESS: THE MODERN-DAY SYNDROME

∂

We all know that stress can be toxic to healthy, glowing skin when unresolved and we have discussed how the stress hormones affect the skin *(see "Your skin and your hormonal health: the complex connection" on page 30-49)*. Typically, untreated stress will rear its ugly head when you're getting ready for that all-important date or you are about to give a presentation and your face lights up like *Rudolph's nose* and there's no hiding it as you suffer the persistent redness of rosacea. Stress can take many forms and often we are so used to being overloaded with tasks, chemicals, work and the demands of modern-day life that we don't even notice that we are stressed. Let me ask you, when you go on holiday do you get sick within two to three days? When you fly, do you get a cold or the flu? Does your skin break out? Does your rosacea get worse with flushing or your skin become itchy? This is your body telling you it is under stress and it is struggling to achieve a healthy balance.

Stress can present in many ways. These generally sit in three categories: mental stress, physical stress and emotional stress.

Mental stress may be seen during periods where you are studying in a new field, learning a new job, meeting the demands of your home life, and taking exams.

Physical stress is more present when you are dehydrated from working or playing in the sun all day, eating nutritionally poor nutrition food such as highly processed foods/fast foods, or limiting your caloric intake for your daily demands when there is not a weight problem — the swings of the highs and lows of blood sugar levels in the body with high-sugar/fructose foods, drinks and sweets.

Emotional stress may be seen as you operate to a very tight schedule and run from one meeting or appointment to another, without taking time to stop, rest or eat. This might also involve ruminating over a problem, worrying about relationships in relation to work, family, personal and with friends. When this occurs constantly and daily you may be overworking your adrenals.

Now, I know that we all experience stress of one sort from time to time as our modern-day lifestyle has it intimately woven into it. However, when your body is unable to return to balance after a restful night's sleep, holiday or weekend away and you continually feel tired, stressed, easily overwhelmed and find you are gaining weight, then these symptoms are letting you know that you are not in balance any more.

Why? Well your adrenal glands *(see "Your adrenal health" on page 34)* affect your metabolic function (your weight, energy levels and mental clarity, the health and blood supply to your skin, hair, nails and organs); your reproductive hormones, including sperm production and menstrual cycle; and your digestive functions, to name a few.

Stress affects the skin through three main systems: your nervous system (your epidermis is full of nerves), your digestive system and your stress response system.

When any of these systems are out of balance they affect the others due to their relationship from conception. *In utero*, the same base cell that transformed into your skin also transformed into a nerve cell as you were developing and your nerve cells have a direct to your digestive cells via the tenth cranial nerve and your sympathetic and parasympathetic nervous system.

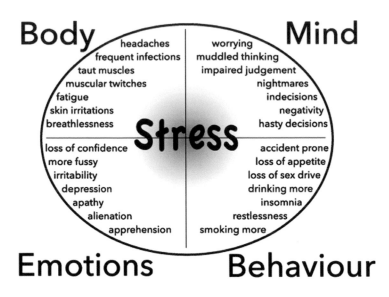

Figure 8: Examples of stress affecting your body, mind, emotions and behaviour

Unmanaged and long-term stress affects your skin, resulting in:

- Dehydrated skin that over- or under-secretes sebum from the sebaceous gland, causing inflammation, blockages and pimples.
- Congestion from sluggish circulation, often presents as milia, as your metabolism slows from fatigue.
- An inability to maintain a healthy pH of 4.5–5.5 as the skin's circulation is reduced and becomes nutrient and oxygen poor.
- Show signs of deterioration such as dullness, infection and/or poor healing, acne that is slow to heal, cold sores, persistent, dry, reddened areas.
- Irritation and flushing such as rosacea, atopic rashes and sun spots from radiation damage.
- Premature ageing such as lines, skin tags (especially around the armpits, chest and neck), dark spots on the face from an increase with free radical damage/inflammation, wrinkles, drooping facial jowls and scarring from skin injuries as well as infections such as resistant acne, cold sores, school sores and insect bites.

Your skin is the mirror to your health. It can reflect your stress levels and how they have influenced your body's health, blood supply and nutrients that may or may not be available for your skin. Imagine your skin, together with the stomach, liver, brain, muscles, heart, and so on, standing in a meal queue to receive its food for the day. Unless the skin is damaged, the skin's place would be at the end of the queue.

Other examples of stressors that are known to affect your adrenal glands are:

- Diet-related factors such as anorexia.
- Emotional stress such as A-type personalities or the death of a family member.
- The stresses of learning a new thing, moving schools, moving house, countries and trying to fit in.
- Regular swimming in a chlorinated pool, working in a fertiliser factory or with chemicals such as hairdressers, nail technicians and painters, a recent move into a brand new home with new carpets, and so on.
- Taking or using steroid creams, inhalants and medications such as the contraceptive pill and antidepressants, antacids, codeine-based pain relief, just to name a few.
- Any major health changes that require intervention, such as an anaesthetic, car accident, surgery, long-term illnesses or long-term antibiotics.

If you can relate to these factors and feel that your energy levels are low, your skin is reactive and slow to heal, then you would benefit from checking the health of your adrenals. The gold standard is a saliva test that involves collecting your saliva four times in one day. Ask your natural practitioner to assist you with this.

Breathing and alchemy

Breathing is essential for life, but when we are stressed and on the run with day-to-day appointments, tasks and activities, we often only breathe shallowly and therefore you do not give your body the oxygen it needs and the opportunity to remove carbon dioxide waste. One of the best ways to improve your breathing and reduce your body's response to stress, no prizes if you guessed what I was going to say in advance, is by exercise! Not only does it encourage you to breathe more deeply, but it also burns up excess adrenaline that has been secreted throughout the day in response to the stressors — which is always a problem if you have a desk job!

The primary role of breathing is to absorb oxygen and expel carbon dioxide through the movement of the lungs. Muscles that control the movement of the lungs are the diaphragm (a sheet of muscle underneath the lungs) and the muscles between the ribs.

When you are under stress your breathing pattern changes.[28] Typically, you will take small, shallow breaths, using your shoulders rather than your diaphragm to move air in and out of your lungs. This style of breathing disrupts the balance of gases in the body.

Shallow over-breathing, or hyperventilation, can prolong feelings of anxiety by making the physical symptoms of stress worse. Controlling your breathing can help to improve some of these symptoms.

Relaxation response

When you are relaxed, you breathe through your nose in a slow, even and gentle way. Deliberately copying a relaxed breathing pattern seems to calm the nervous system that controls the body's involuntary functions.

Controlled breathing can cause physiological changes that include:
- lowered blood pressure and heart rate
- reduced levels of stress hormones in the blood
- reduced lactic acid build-up in muscle tissue
- balanced levels of oxygen and carbon dioxide in the blood
- improved immune system functioning
- increased physical energy
- increased feelings of calm and wellbeing.

Special considerations

Some people find that concentrating on their breathing actually provokes panic and hyperventilation. If this happens to you, look for another way to relax and consider having your thyroid gland checked for its efficiency and your iodine levels too, as this is vital to healthy hormones and when out of balance can contribute to an increased feeling of anxiety.

Abdominal breathing for relaxation

There are different breathing techniques to bring about relaxation. In essence, the general aim is to shift from upper chest breathing to abdominal breathing. You will need a quiet, relaxed environment where you won't be disturbed for 10 to 20 minutes. Set an alarm if you don't want to lose track of time.

Sit comfortably and raise your ribcage to expand your chest. Place one hand on your chest and the other on your abdomen. Take notice of how your upper chest and abdomen are moving while you breathe. Concentrate on your breath and try to gently breathe in and out through the nose. Your upper chest and stomach should be still, allowing the diaphragm to work more efficiently with your abdomen, rather than your chest.

With each exhalation, allow any tension in your body to slip away. Once you are breathing slowly using your abdomen, sit quietly and enjoy the sensation of physical relaxation.

As you can see, it is important to not let stress get the upper hand, so I hope that you will incorporate and enjoy the benefits of introducing regular exercise and breathing techniques into your beauty and health regime.

Another simple strategy that you can implement on a daily basis is by using **alchemy (the science and medicinal benefits of aromatherapy)**. It helps to balance the day's demands and keep your body calm and balanced.

Diffusing oils in your home or place of work is an easy way to keep your frustration level low. My favourite blend for managing the day-to-day stressors uses the following ingredients. I have it at home and at my clinic in a diffuser. This is a great blend to use when you are doing breathing techniques too. You can also rub the blends on your feet or temples when you are out and about.

3 drops of basil

3 drops of rosemary

3 drops of peppermint

3 drops of lemon

If you want to try this blend, make sure that the oils are of therapeutic quality to ensure you get the medicinal benefits.

EXERCISE

❧

As we have touched on previously, we lead a much more sedentary lifestyle now with the way we complete our day-to-day tasks. No longer do we regularly undertake tasks in an arduous and lengthy way, such as washing our clothes by hand, putting them through a wringer, walking 500 metres to the clothes line, hanging them out to dry and then bringing them in when dry to be ironed. Yes, as a child I do remember those days when I used to help my mum. My favourite part was the wringer!

Now our daily tasks have become much more automated, which means a reduction in the need for human energy expenditure, exertion and incidental exercise, resulting in our lives becoming gradually more sedentary. To combat this, we need to find other ways to be active.

Parking further away from the supermarket, taking the stairs instead of the lifts or escalators, and making time to include exercise as part of your life on a daily basis. I have found that a good way to know how active you have been is to get yourself an upgraded pedometer such as a fitbit™, jawbone™ and others. Wearing one of these, which are easy to use and allow you to measure and objectify just how active you have been for the day. It keeps you honest with yourself.

Your mission, should you choose to accept it,
is 10,000 steps per day!

This is a perfect example of how our lifestyle affects our mentally preconceived ideas, plus how our lives have changed. However, the benefits of exercise do not end there as exercise is vital for hormonal health; a great workout or "workout glow" is as good as a facial for promoting healthy skin and our muscles, bones and joints need exercise to keep up active and strong.

Daily exercise dissolves and helps to burn the adrenal hormones cortisol and adrenalin that are released during stressful periods in your body and counterbalances the demands on your other hormones such as oestrogen, progesterone, testosterone, insulin and thyroxine. These hormones, in particular, have a negative, cascading effect on your health, resulting in symptoms such as acne, rosacea, psoriasis and fatigue that drains you of your quality life because you are just too tired. In my clinical experience, when you treat the imbalance in your health, your skin glows.

To paint you a picture, your adrenal hormones are like millions of guerrilla-style soldiers who can't distinguish between the hostiles or friendlies. Adrenal hormones, if not acted upon by exercise/activity, can undermine healthy cells and create a more acidic environment in your body, which leads to other lifestyle diseases such as cardiovascular disease, diabetes and metabolic syndrome.[2]

In discussing exercise we would be remiss if we did not talk about the basic fundamentals of exercise. Some people believe that weight loss and a healthy weight are the result of calories in versus calories out. This means a balance between what you eat and the energy that you expend or burn up. While there is some truth to this, regardless of age it may be an oversimplification as there are many variables to achieving a healthy weight. These are genetics, metabolic health — that is, how healthy your adrenal, thyroid and hormonal health is (as previously discussed) — and dietary influences.

So what other benefits do we get from exercise? Here are some health benefits of exercise that I hope will inspire you to get started and make exercise a crucial and essential part of your everyday lifestyle.

1. Releases beta-endorphins — anti-depressants.

2. Promotes skin health through enhanced circulation as the body uses this medium to control body temperature.

3. Improves hormonal health and insulin resistance, especially PCOS (polycystic ovary syndrome).

4. Releases growth hormone, helps stage III and IV sleep — deep sleep, anti-ageing, hormonal balancing, including blood sugar.[4]

5. Prevents osteoporosis.

6. Increases oxygen to the brain.

7. Lowers cholesterol.

8. Burns fat tissue, especially aerobic sessions over 40 minutes.

9. Helps coronary arteries by enlarging openings.

10. Releases circulating fibrinolysins — keeps blood viscosity down, so you are less likely to have a thrombosis (blood clot).

11. Clears "acidosis" from food allergies.

12. Improves your digestive tract and microbiome family and therefore improving your food breakdown and nutrient recovery and absorption.

13. Strengthens you immune system.

14. Promotes joint mobility.

15. Helps overcome "mental puff/brain fog" — focus and clarity improves.

16. Develops stamina and endurance, especially strength exercise.

17. Purges pesticides and herbicides through sweat ducts, especially effective if your Iodine levels are normal.

18. Enhances libido.

19. Assists in preventing cancer.

20. Improves circulation throughout the whole body, improving physical, emotional and metal clarity — "Ah ha!" memory therefore improves (building flashes of realisation).

21. Improves your energy and self-esteem.

22. Deemed as the safest way to reduce chronic inflammation that causes diabetes, heart disease, memory loss.[3]

So, I guess if you are not doing regular exercise you may be saying to yourself I know I need to incorporate exercise, but how am I going to fit it in?

Whether you divide your exercise/activity up into 10 and 15 minute segments, or do it in one session, everyone will benefit from at least 30–40 minutes of daily exercise at their initial fitness level.

To increase your regular exercise quota, try the following as well as a regular exercise programme for your age, fitness level and current health status:

- Dancing — aerobic dance can burn upwards of 443 calories per hour. And yes, sweaty Saturday-night dance parties totally count.

- Take the stairs, not the escalator or lift — scaling steps can burn almost 300 more calories than running on flat ground. That's 852 calories per hour if you have that many stairs!
- Park the car further away from your destination.
- Walking briskly for up to 40 minutes a day for weight loss.
- Cycling — pedalling on a stationary bike can burn just as many calories as jogging (398 calories) even though you get to sit down while you do it. Dust off your old mountain bike or take a vigorous indoor cycling class, and you'll burn even more calories (both burn about 483 per hour, depending on your speed and resistance).
- Playing golf.
- Swimming — you can't lose with breaststroke (585 calories per hour), backstroke (540 calories per hour), or butterfly (784 calories per hour) at a moderate to vigorous pace.
- Shooting hoops or skipping — your favourite childhood playground game is actually an incredible workout. Depending on your pace and intensity, it can burn about 670 calories an hour. Shoot for at least 100 skips per minute to get the most 'bang' for your bounce.
- Pacing while talking on the phone.
- Walk your dog or a neighbour's dog.
- Walk along the beach and you will get two benefits, as you will be exercising and grounding yourself too.

If you want to measure your energy expenditure in kilojoules, 1 calorie (nutritional) is 4.1868 kilojoules.

As the list above shows, the guidelines don't require meeting the time recommendations through structured exercise alone. Half the time can be spent on structured activity, while the other half can be accumulated from using the stairs or walking around whenever possible (at work, enjoying retail therapy or at home).

Making exercise a priority

Most people can reach the recommended activity/exercise goals by simply making a conscious decision to make it part of their daily routine.

The key to increasing exercise in your day-to-day activity is to make exercise a habit and figure out which time of the day works best as well as looking for ways to increase walking and activity.

Suggested times may be:

- Before going to work.
- During your lunch hour.
- Right after work.
- In the evening with a friend.

Allow yourself to be flexible so you can find out what works for you and then stick to it. Remember, it only takes a month to create a new habit, but it can also be broken easily when you get out of the routine such as during holidays, illness and work travel. So, be mindful and allow yourself to fall off the wagon but then get back on and re-establish your habit. It may not be in your 20s or 30s that you see the benefits as much as when you reach your late 40s, 50s and 60s. It is then that your strong habits will make you who you are and become invaluable. So make your habits beneficial ones!

Weekly food programme

Table 10: Weekly food programme

Breakfast	Lunch	
Hot water with fresh lemon Fruit, nut and seed mix with kefir yoghurt and berries Green tea	Creamy chicken coleslaw	
Hot water with fresh lemon Kefir breakfast	Black rice salad	
Hot water with fresh lemon. Mexican scrambled tofu Green tea	Chicken Waldorf salad	
Carrot juice Kefir breakfast Green tea	Mayan avocado salad	
Hot water with fresh lemon Fruit, nut and seed mix with kefir yoghurt and berries Green tea	Protein-rich tuna salad	
Liver support daily juice 2 boiled eggs with spelt or gluten-free toast Green tea	Healthy chicken burger and baked sweet potato fries	
Hot water with fresh lemon Sensational buckwheat pancakes with fresh berries and cashew cream Green tea	Fresh garden salad with mustard dressing	

Dinner	Snacks and sweet treats	Exercise
Baked fish with almonds	Sweet green smoothie 1 medium green apple	40 minutes' walk
Lamb cutlets with vegetables	Chocolate brownie 1 medium green apple	40 minutes' walk, 10 push-ups and 10 sit-ups
Traditional Italian meatballs	Beetroot dip with 6–8 rice crackers 1 pear	40 minutes' walk
Grilled salmon steaks with dill butter	Fresh fruit tarts	40 minutes' walk, 15 push-ups and 15 sit-ups
Thai green curry with steamed vegetables	Super bliss balls — no more than 2 1 medium green apple	40 minutes' walk
Nut-crusted fish and salad greens	Adrenal beauty booster 1 medium green apple	40 minutes' walk, 10 push-ups and 10 sit-ups
Chicken fajita casserole	Chocolate mousse	Day of rest

Food diary

Day	
Breakfast	
Snack	
Lunch	
Snack	
Dinner	
Diet review and comments including skin changes	

Day	
Breakfast	
Snack	
Lunch	
Snack	
Dinner	
Diet review and comments including skin changes	

Day	
Breakfast	
Snack	
Lunch	
Snack	
Dinner	
Diet review and comments including skin changes	

Day	
Breakfast	
Snack	
Lunch	
Snack	
Dinner	
Diet review and comments including skin changes	

Day	
Breakfast	
Snack	
Lunch	
Snack	
Dinner	
Diet review and comments including skin changes	

Day	
Breakfast	
Snack	
Lunch	
Snack	
Dinner	
Diet review and comments including skin changes	

Day	
Breakfast	
Snack	
Lunch	
Snack	
Dinner	

Diet review and comments including skin changes

Day	
Breakfast	
Snack	
Lunch	
Snack	
Dinner	

Diet review and comments including skin changes

Day	
Breakfast	
Snack	
Lunch	
Snack	
Dinner	

Diet review and comments including skin changes

Day	
Breakfast	
Snack	
Lunch	
Snack	
Dinner	

Diet review and comments including skin changes

Day	
Breakfast	
Snack	
Lunch	
Snack	
Dinner	

Diet review and comments including skin changes

Day	
Breakfast	
Snack	
Lunch	
Snack	
Dinner	

Diet review and comments including skin changes

Day	
Breakfast	
Snack	
Lunch	
Snack	
Dinner	
Diet review and comments including skin changes	

Day	
Breakfast	
Snack	
Lunch	
Snack	
Dinner	
Diet review and comments including skin changes	

Day	
Breakfast	
Snack	
Lunch	
Snack	
Dinner	

Diet review and comments including skin changes

Day	
Breakfast	
Snack	
Lunch	
Snack	
Dinner	

Diet review and comments including skin changes

Day	
Breakfast	
Snack	
Lunch	
Snack	
Dinner	
Diet review and comments including skin changes	

Day	
Breakfast	
Snack	
Lunch	
Snack	
Dinner	
Diet review and comments including skin changes	

Day
Breakfast	
Snack	
Lunch	
Snack	
Dinner	

Diet review and comments including skin changes

Day
Breakfast	
Snack	
Lunch	
Snack	
Dinner	

Diet review and comments including skin changes

Day	
Breakfast	
Snack	
Lunch	
Snack	
Dinner	
Diet review and comments including skin changes	

Day	
Breakfast	
Snack	
Lunch	
Snack	
Dinner	
Diet review and comments including skin changes	

Day	
Breakfast	
Snack	
Lunch	
Snack	
Dinner	

Diet review and comments including skin changes

Day	
Breakfast	
Snack	
Lunch	
Snack	
Dinner	

Diet review and comments including skin changes

RECIPE INDEX

BREAKFAST

Kefir breakfast

Ingredients

2–4 tablespoons Babushka yoghurt

1–2 tablespoons fresh fruit: strawberries, apricots, blueberries, kiwi fruit or whatever is in season

1 teaspoon psyllium husks

¼ teaspoon raw honey

Method

Blend all the ingredients together and eat immediately. To get the full benefit, drink 1 litre of filtered water with lemon 30 minutes prior to breakfast and then 2 hours after.

Fruit, nut and seed mix

Ingredients

1½ cups mixed raw nuts (organic) — almonds, walnuts, cashews, macadamia nuts, hazelnuts, pine nuts, pecans, Brazil nuts, peanuts and pistachios are all great options!

1 cup seeds — pumpkin, sesame, sunflower, chia and flax work well

Optional: 4/6 dates or prunes, or 1 whole apple (to add sweetness)

Optional: ½ cup wheatgerm (to add bulk)

Method

Soak the nuts and seeds overnight (minimum 8 hours). Rinse the nuts thoroughly until the water runs clear. Soak the sesame seeds separately in a sieve, so you do not lose any when rinsing. Blend the nuts together in a blender until roughly chopped, add the seeds and blend again until also roughly chopped. Add dates and/or prunes to the blender and blend once more until roughly chopped. Serve immediately or store in the refrigerator in an airtight container.

To serve

1 tablespoon safflower oil — do not cook as it goes rancid when heated! Coconut yoghurt (COYO brand is good).

Nut milk

Ingredients

3–4 cups filtered water

1 cup nuts (almonds or hazelnuts)

3 dates, agave or honey (optional for extra sweetness)

½ teaspoon vanilla bean extract

Sea or Himalayan sea salt

Note: ¾ cup raw almonds = 1 cup soaked as they expand.

Method

Soak the almonds overnight, for approximately 12 hours. Rinse the nuts thoroughly. Place all the ingredients in a blender and blend them at high speed for approximately 30 seconds. Pour the mixture into a nut milk bag or, if using a blender with a filter, insert the filter and after 4 seconds open the tap to draw the milk into a jug.

Hazelnut chocolate

Hazelnut milk

1 tablespoon cacao

1 tablespoon agave

1–2 frozen bananas

Pina colada

Macadamia milk

1 young coconut

1 cup pineapple

1 cup frozen mango

1 frozen banana

Strawberry cardamom shake

Cashew milk

1 cup strawberries

¼ teaspoon ground cardamom

1 tablespoon honey

Easy tahini milk

2 tablespoons tahini

½ teaspoon vanilla extract

3 cups filtered water — to taste

1½ tablespoons agave — to taste

No soaking or straining required

Sensational buckwheat pancakes

Just when you thought you would never see a pancake again!

Ingredients

½ cup buckwheat

½ cup almond/oat/hazelnut meal

1 tablespoon potato starch

1/8 cup unsweetened oat/soy/rice milk or water to mix

1 egg

Method

Combine all the ingredients in a bowl. In a non-stick pan, cook the pancakes on a moderate heat for approximately 2–3 minutes on each side. If necessary, you can use coconut oil or a small amount of ghee to prevent the pancakes sticking. Watch carefully as they may burn quickly. Try serving with ½ cup mixed berries or stewed apple and cinnamon and cashew cream.

Chicken sausage and sautéed vegetables

A hearty, warm dish, perfect for winter.

Ingredients

2 gluten-free chicken or turkey sausages cut into 1–2 cm slices

1 cup mixed, chopped onion, mushroom and green capsicum

1 cup washed, fresh spinach leaves

Method

Microwave the spinach in a microwave-safe bowl or steam until wilted (3–5 minutes). Chop into bite-sized pieces and place on a plate. Place the chopped vegetables and sausage into a hot oiled pan and sauté until the sausages are cooked through. Spoon the mixture over the spinach. Season with salt and pepper and serve.

Mexican-style scrambled tofu

A modern adaptation from ancient Mexico.

Ingredients

200 g silken tofu

1 cup of any colour tomato, zucchini and onion

1 tablespoon olive oil

1 teaspoon mixed herbs

Tabasco sauce (optional)

Cracked pepper and sea salt to taste

Paprika — to taste

Method

Finely chop the vegetables, add to the oiled fry pan and sauté with the mixed herbs until tender. Add the tofu, breaking up and stirring until heated through. Add 2 drops of Tabasco sauce (optional) and season with salt and pepper to taste. Place on a plate and sprinkle lightly with paprika. Serve with Tabasco sauce on the side.

SMOOTHIES

Sweet green smoothie

Ingredients

1 cup sweet potato leaf/lettuce leaves/bok choy

1 medium-sized silverbeet leaf

1 whole, medium-sized pear

1 banana/pineapple

Freshly cut ginger

½ stick celery (using the leaves is OK)

Honey or liquid stevia or yacón syrup

Super-foods — Maca powder (only if your testosterone is low), Vital Greens, Mila or similar as recommended

300 ml chilled water

Method

Tear up the silverbeet and sweet potato leaves and add then to the blender. Add all the other ingredients followed by the chilled water. Blend all the ingredients until they are the desired consistency.

Adrenal beauty booster

Ingredients

½ small cucumber, chopped

2-3 leaves of kale or spinach (if using kale, blanch a little in hot water prior to blending to promote digestion and to relax the liver — this also helps prevent gas or bloating)

½ small avocado

1 small apple

1 tablespoon lemon juice

1 tablespoon chia seeds

1 tablespoon Maca powder

5 fresh mint leaves

A pinch of cinnamon

1 teaspoon grated ginger (optional)

Method

Measure out all the ingredients and blend together, then enjoy.

JUICES

Whole lemon zinger

Makes two glasses.

Ingredients

1 medium-sized lemon

Honey or liquid stevia (NuNaturals Liquid Stevia will give you zero calories and zero GI)

Iced water makes a refreshing summer drink OR use warm water for a soothing, hot drink in winter.

Method

Place the whole lemon in your blender. Add the water until it is halfway up or to the top of the lemon, depending on your taste preference. Finally, add the honey or Liquid stevia to suit your taste and blend. If your blender has a tap, wait 10 seconds and turn on the tap to enjoy a fresh lemon zinger.

Carrot juice

Ingredients

2 medium carrots

500 ml filtered water

1 medium lemon

1 tablespoon ginger

2 small sticks celery

Method

Using a juicer or filter in a blender, mix together all the ingredients and drink immediately.

Liver support daily juice

Ingredients

¼ medium beetroot

3 small carrots

½ grapefruit

1 green apple

2 tablespoons lemon juice — to taste

1 cm square fresh ginger

Method

Using a juicer or filter in a blender, mix together all the ingredients and drink immediately. Makes approximately 300 ml.

SOUPS

Creamy dill and cauliflower soup

Ingredients

1 tablespoon of organic coconut oil or ghee

1 large onion, chopped

4–6 cloves of garlic chopped (or to taste)

1 large head or two small heads of cauliflower, cuts into chunks

Handful of cauliflower florets, separated from the cauliflower head

6 tablespoons fresh or 2 tablespoons of dried dill

4–6 cups of water

Sea salt to taste

Method

In a large pot, melt the ghee or coconut oil and add dill. Add onion and sauté until translucent. Add garlic and sauté for a few minutes. Add cauliflower chunks and dill if using fresh and enough water to cover. Simmer until tender, then puree in a blender and return it to the pot. Add approximately 4 cups of filtered water, depending on desired thickness. Add sea salt to taste and the florets. Simmer until tender. Variation: Use chicken stock instead of filtered water.

Beetroot soup with beans

Ingredients

2 tablespoons olive oil

1 medium onion, thinly sliced

3 medium beetroot, grated

3 medium carrots, grated

1 yellow capsicum, cored and chopped

4 medium tomatoes, chopped

1 litre/4 cups vegetable stock

5 cups filtered water

440 g black beans, drained and rinsed

1 teaspoon garlic powder or 2 fresh cloves

Sea salt and black pepper to taste

¼ lemon

2 handfuls chopped parsley

Method

In a large pot, heat the olive oil over a medium heat. Add the onion and cook, stirring occasionally, until the onion is translucent, for about 4 minutes. Add the beetroot, carrots, capsicum and tomatoes. Cover and cook, stirring occasionally, until the vegetables start to soften, for about 5 to 7 minutes. Add the vegetable stock, water, black beans and garlic powder or cloves. Season with salt and pepper and bring to the boil. Reduce the heat. Cover and cook for about 10 minutes. Squeeze the lemon juice into the soup and drop the squeezed lemon piece into the soup too. Add the parsley. Cook the soup for another 2 to 3 minutes and turn off the heat. Serve with 1 to 2 tablespoons kefir yoghurt or cashew cheese.

Easy pumpkin soup with cashew cream

Ingredients

500 g Jap pumpkin

2 litres chicken stock

3 cloves fresh garlic

2 medium potatoes

2 carrots

2 red onions

Salt, pepper and nutmeg to taste

Method

Prepare all the ingredients and place in a large pot and cook for approximately 30 minutes or until all the vegetables are soft. Blend all the ingredients until smooth and creamy. Add salt and pepper to taste. When serving, add a sprinkle of nutmeg and serve with a teaspoon of cashew cheese in the centre of the bowl.

Old-fashioned vegetable soup

Ingredients

3 cloves garlic

2 medium carrots

4 sticks celery

2 sweet potatoes

2 medium red onions

2 medium zucchini

200 g pumpkin

1 cup of pearl barley

2 litre of chicken stock/a ham hock/a lamb shank, depending on your preference

Salt and pepper to taste

Method

Prepare and place all the vegetables, cut into 1 cm cubes, together with the garlic and barley into a large pot together with the chicken stock/ham hock/lamb shank and add salt and pepper. Place on a slow heat and allow to cook for 1 ½–2 hours or until the meat is cooked. Remove ham hock or lamb shank if used Allow it to cool and remove any excess fat. Reheat and serve immediately.

DIPS

Pumpkin dip with quinoa salad

Ingredients

250 g butternut pumpkin, seeds and skin removed

1 clove garlic

1½ teaspoons cumin

1 tablespoon cashew paste

¼ cup white quinoa

1 bunch chopped parsley — to taste

1 small red onion

3 tablespoons extra virgin olive oil

150 g green beans

½ punnet cherry tomatoes

½ bunch radish, quartered

2 lemons

Pita or mountain bread to your liking

Method

Cut the pumpkin into 2 cm cubes and steam until soft and tender then set aside to cool. When cool, place the pumpkin in a food processor with the garlic, cumin, cashew paste, olive oil and juice of half a lemon. Season with salt and pepper, and blend until it is smooth then set it aside. Meanwhile, cook the quinoa in 1 cup of boiling water for 12–15 minutes. Rinse well under cold water, drain and set it aside. In a small bowl, mix the cooked quinoa with the onion, parsley juice of half a lemon, salt and pepper, drizzle with olive oil and mix well. Blanche the green beans in boiling water for 1 minute then refresh in cold water. Arrange the dip and quinoa salad on a large platter. Serve with green beans, radish and cherry tomatoes, wedges of lemon and pita or mountain bread.

Beetroot dip

Ingredients

1 medium beetroot

½–¾ cup walnuts

1 clove garlic — to taste

Juice from ½–1 lime

4-8 dates or ½ teaspoon yacón syrup

Parsley

Tahini — to taste

Salt and pepper

Method

Pulse the garlic and herbs in a blender then add the remaining ingredients and process to the desired consistency.

Quick and easy guacamole

Ingredients

2 avocados

1 tomato, seeds removed

Juice from a small lemon

½ Spanish onion

¼ cup coriander

Thai sweet chilli sauce

Himalayan salt and pepper

Method

Cut the tomato in half and remove the seeds then dice in to small but not fine pieces. Blend the coriander and the Spanish onion together until the desired consistency has been reached. Cut the avocados in half and remove the skin and seeds then place in the blender with the onion and coriander. Squeeze in the lemon juice and add salt, pepper and Thai sweet chilli sauce to taste. Do a taste test and serve with dipping vegetables and breads of your choice.

SIDES AND SUPPORTS

Baked sweet potato fries

Ingredients

3 large sweet potatoes, peeled and cut into wedges

1 tablespoon walnut or coconut oil

½ teaspoon sea salt

½--1 teaspoon cinnamon

¼ teaspoon paprika

Method

Preheat the oven to 220° Celsius. In a mixing bowl, toss all the ingredients (except the cinnamon) until the potato wedges are evenly coated with the oil and spices. Place on a baking sheet, separated evenly, and then sprinkle the cinnamon on top as desired. Bake for 30 minutes or until golden-brown.

Cashew cream

Ingredients

1 cup organic, raw cashews, soaked for 8 hours to activate

¼–½ cup filtered water depending on desired thickness

1–2 tablespoons maple syrup, or yacón syrup — to taste

½ teaspoon natural vanilla extract, or a little more — to taste

A pinch of Celtic sea salt

Method

Place all the ingredients into the blender and puree until thick and creamy. It is a good idea to start with the ¼ cup of water, and then gradually thin it out in order to achieve your desired thickness.

**Please note: you will need a high-speed blender, such as a Vitamix or Thermomix to achieve a really creamy consistency. With a conventional blender, you must soak the cashews by covering them with room temperature water for about 4 hours or the quick way (albeit not raw) by covering with boiling water for 15 minutes.

Roast vegetable salad

Ingredients

2 medium sweet potatoes (may also use plain)

1 medium sized beetroot

250 g pumpkin

2 medium-sized carrots

2 tablespoons extra virgin coconut oil

I tablespoon mayonnaise

Organic dried paprika to sprinkle over the vegetables

Method

Cut all the vegetables into 2 cm cubes except the beetroot, which should be cut into 1 cm cubes. Place them into a container or plastic bag together with the coconut oil and paprika and mix thoroughly until all pieces are coated.

Place in a moderate oven at 180° Celsius for 15–20 minutes or until cooked. Place them into a serving bowl with the mayonnaise and mix through. Serve immediately with fish, chicken or lamb.

Cauliflower rice

You will need a blender/mixer for this recipe.

Ingredients

1 medium apple

1 medium cauliflower

1 medium onion

2 gloves of garlic

1 piece of fresh ginger, approximately 2 cm cube

1 medium zucchini

2 carrots

2 teaspoons curry powder

1 teaspoon turmeric

1 teaspoon ground cumin

2/3 cup coconut cream

1 tablespoon cornflour, unbleached

Salt and pepper to taste

Filtered water

1 tablespoon coconut oil

Method

Place garlic, ginger and spices in the blender and mix. Add the apple, cauliflower, carrots, onion and zucchini and mix until it has the consistency of rice.

Prepare a hot wok and add 1 tablespoon of coconut oil for cooking. Add the rice-like mixture and cook on a high heat for 10 minutes. Decrease the heat, add 2/3 cup of coconut cream and continue to cook for a further 10 minutes or until cooked. Lastly, mix the cornflour with filtered water and add to the rice mixture until it thickens. Cook for a further minute and add salt and pepper to taste

Serve with your favourite meat.

LIGHT MEALS

Healthy chicken burger

Ingredients

500 g lean chicken mince

1 egg, lightly beaten

1 tablespoon dried sage

1 lemon, grated zest and juice

1-2 tablesppons Coconut oil

1 large red onion

¼ cup seasoned potato flour

8 slices bread or hamburger rolls (preferably sourdough)

½ cup of whole egg mayonnaise

50 g mixed salad leaves

Method

Combine the mince, egg, sage and lemon zest in a bowl. Season and mix well. Shape into 4 even-sized patties, cover and chill for 20 minutes. Heat 1 teaspoon of coconut oil in a frying pan on medium. Sauté the onion for 2–3 minutes or until transparent, stirring occasionally. Remove the onion from the pan and cover to keep warm. Heat 1 teaspoon of coconut oil in the same pan. Dust the patties in seasoned potato flour, shaking off any excess. Slightly flatten the patties and place them in the pan. Cook on a medium heat for 4–6 minutes on each side or until golden and cooked through. Drain on paper towel. Squeeze lemon juice over the patties. Spread the bread/rolls with mayonnaise, add 4 slices of salad leaves and some onion and place the patties on top with the remaining leaves

Variation: Replace the bread for gluten-free/quinoa/buckwheat or spelt flour bread.

San choy bow (pork mince in lettuce cups)

Ingredients

325 g pork fillet, minced

1 cup sliced water chestnuts, drained

1 tablespoon sliced ginger

1 tablespoon chilli sauce

2 tablespoons sherry

1 tablespoons tamari or soy sauce

Iceberg lettuce leaves, cut carefully into cups

Method

Sauté the sliced ginger lightly before browning the pork mince. Add sherry and sauces with water chestnuts and simmer for five minutes. Thin with a little water. Spoon the mixture into lettuce cups to serve. Serve with mixed, steamed Chinese vegetables.

Soy and garlic kebabs

Served cold, these are the ultimate ready-to-eat healthy snack.

Ingredients

180 g chicken or lean lamb, cut into cubes

1 cup onion and green capsicum, cut into wedges

1 cup cherry tomatoes

2 tablespoons garlic, crushed

Chilli to taste (optional)

3 tablespoons soy sauce

A pinch of salt

Cracked black pepper

Method

Soak wooden skewers in water for ½ hour so they do not burn. Pierce the cubed chicken/lamb, onion, green capsicum and cherry tomatoes on to the skewers. Mix the garlic, soy and seasoning in a small bowl and brush the kebabs with the mixture. Cook, in a pan, BBQ or under the grill until the chicken is cooked through. Serve with a salad or vegetables or keep cold in fridge as a snack.

Garlic and soy chicken drumsticks

Ingredients

6 chicken drumsticks

3 tablespoons soy sauce

1 tablespoon crushed garlic

Coconut oil for cooking

Method

Cook the drumsticks with garlic and soy in a covered pan on a low heat until cooked through. Turn regularly. These may be served cold.

Lemon chicken nibbles

An excellent meal that can be cooked in less than 15 minutes.

Ingredients

½ cup lemon juice

1 tablespoon salt-reduced soy sauce

1 tablespoon French or spicy mustard

1 teaspoon olive oil

A pinch of cayenne pepper

180 g chicken breasts, diced

Method

Combine the lemon juice, soy sauce, mustard, olive oil and cayenne pepper. Add the diced chicken and toss around in a bowl to coat the pieces well. Leave to marinate for an hour or so if you wish. Heat the pan and fry the chicken. Halfway through frying, turn the chicken over and marinate with more sauce. Cook this side for a further 10 minutes or until cooked. Serve with a salad.

Note: Chicken can also be grilled or placed on a BBQ.

SALADS

Mayan avocado salad

Ingredients

½ avocado

1 large plate of mixed salad greens and sprouts

6–8 king prawns (or 150 g) with a squeeze of lemon

OR

1 cup Vegusto cheese (or 120 g), chopped shallots and a pinch of cayenne pepper

Juice of ½ a lime

Method

Cover the plate of greens with either the cheese or prawns. Garnish with thin slices of avocado and dress with the lime juice.

*Vegusto cheese can be found in most health food shops and is made from non-hydrogenised vegetable oils and fats (coconut, canola), potato starch, fruit juice, rice flour, yeast, nut butter (100% almonds), rock salt, flavouring (vegetable), binder (carrageen), spices, antioxidant (ascorbic acid), colourants (turmeric, beta-carotene). It is garlic-free.

Chicken Caesar salad

One of the most popular salad recipes.

Ingredients

90 g chicken breast, cut into pieces

1 poached egg

1 tablespoon lemon juice

1 tablespoon water

1 teaspoon cracked black pepper

1 teaspoon coconut oil

2 tablespoons traditional mayonnaise

1 cup cos lettuce

Anchovies (optional)

Method

Heat a fry pan with coconut oil if not non-stick. Cook the chicken pieces till brown then remove the chicken from the heat and allow it to cool. Mix together the lemon juice, mayonnaise, warm water, oil and pepper in a bowl. Place the salad greens, chicken and egg in a bowl. Pour the salad dressing over the salad and dress with anchovies (if used).

Fresh garden salad

A light, crisp and easy to prepare salad.

Ingredients

180 g chicken

¼ cup sliced celery

¼ cup sliced red capsicum

¼ cup fresh snow peas

1 cup lettuce

1 avocado, sliced

1 small tomato, cut into wedges

1 lemon, squeezed

Cracked black pepper

1 tablespoon low-carbohydrate mayonnaise

1 tablespoon extra virgin olive oil

Method

Combine all the ingredients together and dress with the mustard dressing.

Mustard dressing

1½ teaspoons Dijon mustard

100 ml cold pressed olive oil

50 ml freshly squeezed lemon juice

Method

Place all the dressing ingredients into a container and shake well to combine. Add extra olive oil to taste. Drizzle over the salad and serve immediately.

Chicken Waldorf salad

Ingredients

200 g steamed chicken fillet, chopped

½ cup green apple, chopped

½ cup celery, chopped

6 walnuts

Red onion to taste

2 tablespoons mayonnaise

Method

Combine all ingredients, season with pepper and sea salt and serve.

Mediterranean salad

Ingredients

1 cup salad greens — include bitter greens such as rocket or watercress

1 hard-boiled egg

Slices of red onion and cucumber

125 g can tuna or salmon

4 black olives (optional)

Method

Combine all the ingredients. Dress the salad with one dessertspoon extra virgin olive oil and sprinkle with vinegar (apple cider, red wine or balsamic) or lemon juice.

Optional extras to add variety: Blanched green beans, asparagus, anchovies, ¼ avocado, 1 artichoke, feta, mixed herbs, oven-roasted capsicum or eggplant strips, marinated mushrooms.

Protein-rich tuna salad

Ingredients

1 95 g can tuna (or 90 g fresh)

1 whole egg

1 cup mixed, shredded lettuce, celery rings, shallots, parsley and thinly sliced fresh mushrooms

1 teaspoon sesame seeds

Sprinkling of French herbs or herbs of your choice

Squeeze of lemon juice

Freshly ground black pepper

Olive oil

Method

Shallow fry the sesame seeds until lightly browned, then put aside to cool. Add the olive oil to a non-stick fry pan. Break up the tuna in a small mixing bowl. Mix with the egg and a dash of black pepper. Cook the tuna mix over a moderate heat for 8–10 minutes. Stir frequently, breaking up the larger clumps until light golden brown and flaky. Set aside to cool. Prepare the salad in a small bowl. Drizzle with olive oil and add a squeeze of lemon juice and a sprinkling of French herbs. Gently toss the cooled flaky tuna into the salad and sprinkle with toasted sesame seeds.

Creamy chicken coleslaw

Ingredients

Steamed chicken breast (200 g), finely sliced

2 cups finely chopped cabbage, lightly cooked in boiling water for 5 minutes then rinsed and cooled, finely chopped red onion and grated carrot (you may also substitute with 2 cups of Kim Chi)

¼ cup chopped parsley and chives

2 tablespoons crushed walnuts (optional)

2 tablespoons mayonnaise

Method

Combine all the ingredients in a bowl, mix thoroughly and serve.

Black rice salad

Ingredients

2 cups black rice or quinoa

3 medium-size sweet potatoes (you may also substitute with red potato or Japanese pumpkin)

4 cups chopped kale (soak in water that has boiled, for 5 minutes, drain and dry with paper towel)

3 diced, ripe avocados

Fresh corn off the cob

Diced red onion

Finely diced red chilli

Dill (fresh or dried)

To serve

Macadamia oil (do not cook)

Method

Heat the oven to 180° Celsius.

Rinse and sort the rice, removing any debris. Soak the rice for at least 8 hours or overnight. Rinse and drain. Cook the rice per the instructions on the packet, which is normally 2 cups water to 1 cup rice. Bring to a boil and simmer, covered for about 30 minutes. Remove the cover and fluff the rice then let it cool to room temperature.

Wash, peel and cut your sweet potatoes into small cubes. Lay them out on a lined baking pan evenly. Coat them ever so lightly with olive oil and season with salt pepper and generously with dill (fresh or dried). Bake at 180° Celsius for 30 minutes. Let the sweet potato cool to room temperature. Toss the rice two or three times while the sweet potato is cooking to help it cool.

Once the rice and sweet potato are cooled, transfer them both to a large bowl and mix in the kale, red onion, chilli and avocado. Drizzle in about 2 tablespoons of macadamia oil and season with sea salt, pepper, dill and lemon juice. Mix well, transfer to a clean serving bowl and serve.

Traditional Italian meatballs

Ingredients

500 g lean beef mince

Pepper and salt to taste

4 cloves of garlic, finely chopped or 2 tablespoons pre-minced.

1 egg

1 large onion, diced

4 tablespoons mixed herbs

1 dessertspoon extra virgin coconut oil

Method

Heat the oil in a frying pan. Mix all the remaining ingredients in a large mixing bowl. Shape into small, evenly sized balls and fry in the pan until cooked through. Place them on kitchen paper towels to drain when done. Serve with sauce of your choice and salad or vegetables.

Grilled pepper steak with French beans and lemon butter sauce

Ingredients

2 sirloin or fillet steaks (135 g each)

2 tablespoons extra virgin olive oil

Freshly ground black pepper

2 cups French or green beans

Lemon butter sauce

60 g unsalted ghee

Juice of half a freshly squeezed lemon, freshly squeezed

Freshly ground black pepper

Method

Brush the steaks with olive oil on both sides and season liberally with black pepper. Place under a hot grill, at least 8 cm from the heat, and grill to taste. While the steaks are grilling/cooking, steam the beans until tender but still firm. Heat the ghee in a small saucepan, stir in the lemon juice and freshly ground pepper to taste, and serve over the beans

---

Veal escalopes with a side salad

A delicious way to serve tender veal.

Ingredients

250 g veal mince

1 egg

1 cup spring salad mix

1 clove garlic, crushed

1 lemon — all the juice and half the grated rind

Sea salt, cracked pepper, Italian herbs and Tabasco sauce to desired taste

1 sprig of fresh chopped rosemary

1 tablespoon chopped shallots

2 tablespoons water

Olive oil

Method

Bind together the veal mince, garlic, egg, lemon juice and lemon rind with a sprinkling of Italian herbs, sea salt and pepper. Form into small balls of equal size. Let stand in a cool place for 1 hour. Roll out to a thickness of 1 cm (½ inch thick). Heat the pan, cook the escalopes each on both sides until golden brown. When cooked, remove escalopes from the pan. In the same hot pan, add the chopped shallots, rosemary, Tabasco sauce and water. Stir for a few seconds then pour over the escalopes. Lightly coat the salad mix with hemp seed oil, add a squeeze of lemon juice and a sprinkling of Italian herbs and serve.

Note: Veal mince can be replaced with chicken, turkey, beef or lamb mince.

Nut-crusted fish and salad greens

Ingredients

2 tablespoons extra virgin coconut oil

2 tablespoons unsalted ghee

1/3 cup finely chopped nuts (can be bought or done in a coffee grinder)

1 teaspoon Celtic sea salt

Black pepper to taste

2 large pieces (195 g) of boneless fish, any type will do

2 teaspoons fresh chopped parsley (optional)

2 cups salad greens

1 lemon

Method

Preheat the oven to 220° Celsius. Grease a baking sheet. Melt coconut oil and ghee in a pan. Remove from the heat and leave to cool. Mix the chopped nuts together with the seasoning and put on a plate. Dip the fish in the oil and ghee mixture and then the nut mixture, pressing firmly so the nuts hold. Place the fish on the baking sheet and bake until cooked through. Garnish with fresh parsley. Serve with salad greens, dressed with olive oil and balsamic vinegar, and add a wedge of lemon.

Lamb cutlets with vegetables

Ingredients

180 g of lean lamb cutlets (or beef or veal cutlets)

1 cup cauliflower and broccoli florets

1 teaspoon Worcestershire sauce

½ teaspoon tarragon vinegar

¼ teaspoon onion powder

¼ teaspoon French mustard

2 tablespoons water

Sea salt and freshly ground pepper

Fresh chopped parsley and chives

1 teaspoon slivered almonds

2 tablespoons hemp seed oil

Method

Steam the cauliflower and broccoli florets on a low heat, until tender. Mix the Worcestershire sauce, vinegar, onion powder, mustard, sea salt and pepper with the water. Baste each side of the cutlets with the sauce mixture. Then coat each side lightly with the hemp seed oil. Place under a preheated griller and grill each side until cooked. Serve with cauliflower and broccoli florets.

Grilled salmon steaks with dill butter sauce on a bed of fresh rocket

Ingredients

2 salmon steaks (195 g each)

2 tablespoons olive oil

2 cups of rocket leaves (or mesclun mix)

Dill butter sauce

60 g unsalted ghee

Juice from half a freshly squeezed lemon

2 tablespoons dried or chopped fresh dill

Method

Brush both sides of the salmon with olive oil and grill under high heat for 3-4 minutes per side. Salmon is cooked when the meat is just starting to fall apart. To make the sauce, heat the ghee in a small saucepan, stir in the lemon juice and add the dill. Spread the rocket over a dinner plate, place the salmon on top, cover it with the warm sauce and enjoy immediately.

Baked fish with toasted almonds

Ingredients

325 g trout, salmon or other choice of fish

3/4 cup vegetable mix — green beans, broccoli florets, zucchini

¼ cup onions, thinly sliced

2/3 cup vegetable stock

1 tablespoon fresh chopped fresh parsley

1 small clove garlic, crushed

1 teaspoon almonds, slivered, toasted

Chopped marjoram

Coconut oil

Sea salt

Vinaigrette

1 teaspoon Dijon mustard

1 clove garlic, crushed

4 tablespoons extra virgin olive oil

1 tablespoon balsamic vinegar

1 tablespoon chopped capers

1 tablespoon fresh chopped fresh parsley

4 tablespoons hot water

Method

Steam the green vegetables till tender, strain and put aside to cool. In a fry pan, lightly toast the slivered almonds until golden and put aside to cool.

Vinaigrette: Put all the vinaigrette ingredients in a closed jar and shake it vigorously for a few minutes. Pour the vinaigrette over the vegetables and leave to stand so it soaks into the vegetables — about 25 minutes.

Fish: Clean, wash and dry the fish. Coat a shallow casserole dish with coconut oil. Add the garlic and onions and fry gently until the onion is soft and golden. Place the fish on top of the onion mixture, pour over the vegetable stock then sprinkle with the parsley, marjoram and sea salt. Bake in a preheated oven at 200° Celsius until cooked (up to 25 minutes), basting a few times. Serve garnished with the toasted slivered almonds and green vegetable mix, strained from the vinaigrette.

Chicken fajita casserole

Any choice of meats could replace the chicken.

Ingredients

2 tablespoons coconut oil

500 g chicken breast, cut in strips

2 tablespoons paprika

1 tablespoon turmeric

Salt, pepper, garlic powder, to taste

½ cup onions, thinly sliced

1 cup red and green capsicum strips

½ cup tomato salsa

100 g mixed toasted sesame and pumpkin seeds and crushed pistachio nuts

Method

Preheat the fry pan with the oil and brown the chicken. Stir in the paprika, turmeric, garlic powder, salt and pepper. When the chicken is browned, remove it from the pan and place it in a casserole dish. Add the onions and capsicums to the fry pan and cook for a few minutes until crisp-tender then add to the chicken in the casserole dish. Spread the salsa on top and sprinkle with toasted seed mix. Cook in the oven at 180° Celsius heat for approximately 30 minutes or until tender.

Thai green curry with steamed vegetables

Ingredients

1 chicken breast (200 g)

1 tablespoon extra virgin coconut oil

Green curry paste (no added sugar)

1 medium red onion

Finely chopped ginger to taste

165 ml can coconut milk or cream

2 cups lightly steamed broccoli, beans and zucchini (cut length ways)

Method

Cut the chicken breast into strips, slice onion into rings and sauté together with ginger in coconut oil until the chicken is just cooked. Add coconut milk and green curry paste. Simmer for 5–10 minutes or until cooked. Serve with steamed vegetables.

Thai red curry fish with lime and Asian vegetables

Ingredients

2 medium-size white fish fillets (135 g each)

Red curry paste (no added sugar)

2 tablespoons olive oil for cooking

2 cups bean sprouts, broccoli, onion rings or cabbage strips

1 tablespoon sesame oil

Squeeze of fresh lime juice

Method

Heat the oil in a fry pan. Cut the fish into small portions, about the size of half the palm of your hand. Rub the fish with the red curry paste so it is lightly coated. Shallow fry the fish lightly on both sides. While the fish is cooking, lightly steam the vegetables until tender. Put the mixed vegetables on a plate, top with the sesame oil and lime juice. Serve the fish to one side of the vegetables.

South American chicken salsa

Warm, Mexican-style dish.

Ingredients

180g skinless chicken breast chopped and pounded into thin, bite-size pieces

1 cup mixed broccoli florets and finely sliced green capsicum

1 cup mushrooms, finely sliced

1–2 cloves garlic

2 teaspoons tomato paste

½ cup water

1 teaspoon dried onion flakes or half small red onion, chopped finely

Tabasco sauce, to taste

Sea salt and cracked pepper, to taste

Coconut oil for cooking

Sprinkling of Italian seasoning

Garnish

Fresh chopped parsley and 45 g toasted sunflower, pumpkin and sesame seeds.

Method

Mix together the water, tomato paste, Tabasco sauce, sea salt, pepper and onion flakes (or onion) and leave it to stand. Coat the fry pan with coconut oil and leave to stand. Over a moderate heat, add the crushed garlic, chicken, mushrooms, broccoli and green capsicum. Keep mixing and tossing until the chicken is browned, then add the tomato salsa mixture, stirring well until evenly mixed through. When ready to serve, sprinkle with the garnish.

SWEET TREATS

Fresh fruit tarts

Ingredients

1½ cups almond pulp

1½ cup dates

½ cup desiccated coconut or flour to make the mixture drier if too moist

1½ cups fruit such as apricots, raspberries, plums or whatever fruit is in season

1–2 teaspoons of agave or stevia to taste.

½ teaspoon vanilla

Method

Mix the almond pulp and coconut or flour and press the mixture into the base of a cupcake tray then place this in the fridge whilst preparing the filling. Combine the fruit, vanilla and sweetener together in a blender. Spoon the fruit mixture onto the base in the cupcake tray and place in the fridge again. Add fresh cashew cream on top, immediately before serving *(see recipe on page 143)*

Chocolate brownies

Ingredients

1½ cups almond pulp

1½ cups dates

1½ cups desiccated coconut or flour, to make the mixture drier

¾ cup cocoa

½ cup agave or sweetener, to taste

½ teaspoon vanilla

Optional extras

Sultanas

Sesame seeds

Goji berries or cranberries

Pecans, macadamias and hazelnuts

Method

Combine all the ingredients together. Try not to blend too long as the mixture will become stickier the more it is blended. Put onto baking paper and roll flat using a rolling pin, then score into squares, or make into balls. Place the brownies in the freezer to set.

Chocolate mousse

Ingredients

2 ripe avocados

1/3 cup agave

1/3 cup cacao powder

1 teaspoon vanilla extract

Pinch of salt

Method

Mix all the ingredients together in a bowl until smooth — either by hand or using a stick mixer. Serve immediately or keep refrigerated in an airtight container.

Superfood bliss balls

Preparation time: 5 minutes

Yield: Makes 20+ bites

Ingredients

1½ cups pitted dates

¼ cup organic cocoa nibs

¼ cup shelled hemp hearts

1/3 cup ground flax

¼ cup chia seeds

¼ cup flax seeds

½ cup unsweetened coconut

2 tablespoons virgin coconut oil

Method

Place all the ingredients in the food processor and blend until it forms a smooth dough. If your dates are too dry, you may need to add a couple of tablespoons of warm water. Remove from the food processor and roll into 3–4 centimetre balls and place in the fridge. Store in an airtight container.

Butter mints for sugar cravings

Makes about 64 small butter mints. Serving size: 3–4 butter mints

Packed with healthy, blood-sugar-balancing fats, these butter mints instantly stop sugar cravings and satisfy your sweet tooth while filling you up for hours. You won't believe it until you try it!

Ingredients (dairy-free)

½ cup coconut butter

½ cup coconut oil, liquefied

3 tablespoons raw honey

10–12 drops peppermint essential oil or ¼ teaspoon peppermint extract

2 tablespoons cocoa, if you desire a chocolate flavour

Method

Make sure the coconut butter is at room temperature — it should be soft or slightly runny. If it is solid, place the jar in a saucepan of hot water and stir until it is liquid. Combine all the ingredients. Alternatively, use a spoon to drop small dollops of the mixture onto a parchment-lined baking sheet. Chill until solid.

The dos and don'ts of food

Table 11: Foods to avoid and beneficial foods

Foods to avoid
Dairy — including cheese, butter, milk, cream, yoghurt, ice cream
Trans fats — deep-fried foods and hydrogenated fats such as margarine
Wheat/gluten — If you do choose to eat grains choose organic whole-grain breads and flour. Grind you own grain, if possible. Look for the "no bromine" or "bromine-free" label on commercial baked goods
High-fructose corn syrup (HFCS) 42,55,90
Flavour enhancers — monosodium glutamate (MSG) 621
Preservatives — benzoates 210, 211, 212, 213; nitrates 249, 250, 251, 252; sulphites 220, 221, 222, 223, 224, 225 and 228
Reduce your potato intake and choose sweet potato over white
Food colourings — tartrazine 102; yellow 2G107; sunset yellow FCF110; cochineal 120
Artificial sweetener — aspartame 951

Beneficial Foods		
Vegetables (Carbohydrates)		
Alfalfa sprouts	Chard	Onions
Avocado	Corn	Parsnip
Artichoke	Cucumber	Peas
Asian greens	Eggplant	Pumpkin
Baby spinach	Endives	Radicchio
Bamboo shoots	Fennel	Rocket
Broccoli	Kale	Sea vegetables
Brussels sprouts	Kohlrabi*	Spinach
Cabbage (cooked)	Leeks	Sprouts
Capsicum	Lettuce	fermented
Carrots	Mushrooms	vegetables such
Cauliflower	Okra**	as Kim Chi &
Celery	Olives	sauerkraut

*Kohlrabi is actually pretty fantastic raw! It has a super-crisp texture and a mild, peppery bite

**Okra are small and slender, five-sided pods. They are bright green in colour, with small caps and tapered ends. Inside, their white flesh contains lots of small, edible, white seeds, and it has a mild, zucchini-like flavour

Beneficial Foods continued

Fruit (carbohydrates)

Apples — green are best	Lemons	Peaches
Apricots	Limes	Pears
Blackberries	Mulberries	Raspberries
Cherries	Nectarines	Strawberries
Grapefruit	Passionfruit	Watermelon

Nuts

Almonds	Hazelnuts	Walnuts
Brazil	Macadamia	Seeds — sesame, sunflower, pumpkin, flax
Coconut meat	Pecans	

Beans/Legumes (Only If Vitamin D levels above 75 Nmol)

Black beans	Kidney beans	Lima beans

Proteins

Chicken	Lamb	Scallops
Duck	Mussels	Squid
Eggs	Oysters	Tofu or tempeh/tempe
Fish	Pork*	Turkey
Kangaroo	Prawns	Veal

*including low-cured meat such as bacon and ham

Oils — should be cold-pressed

Apricot kernel	Hemp seed — great for making your own bread	Olive
Coconut — best for cooking		Sesame — great in salad dressings
Flaxseed — high in omega-3	Macadamia — high in omega-9 and great for balancing blood sugar	Walnut — high in omega-3

Dairy

Ghee — the milk solids are removed

Kefir — the beneficial bacteria eat the milk solids and growth factor, making it safe for ingestion

Condiments

Soy sauce	All spices	All herbs

Beneficial Foods				
Grains				
Barley	buckwheat kennels	Oats	Quinoa	Wild or long rice

Foods to increase your daily fiber intake			
apples	bananas	lentils	oats
artichoke	beans	linseeds	onion
asparagus	garlic	nuts	Psylliumhusks

Omega-3

Found in oils such as canola, flax, soybean

Nuts: walnuts

Fish: oily fish — herring, mackerel, salmon, trout and tuna

Other: algae, eggs

Omega-6

Found in oils such as canola, corn, olive, peanut, safflower, soybean and sunflower

Nuts: almonds, cashews, hazelnuts, peanuts, pecans, pistachios and walnuts

Other: eggs

Omega-9

Found in oils such as canola, olive, peanut, safflower, sunflower

Nuts: almonds, cashews, hazelnuts, macadamias, peanuts, pecans, pistachios, walnuts

Other: avocado, eggs, poultry

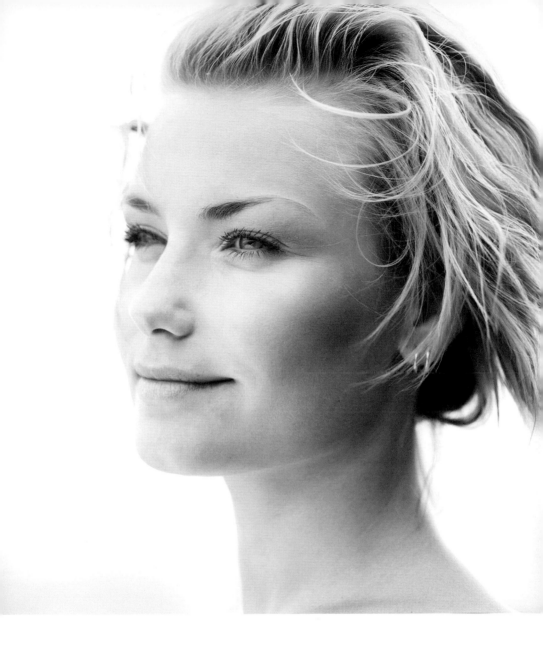

SECTION
THREE

Sections One and Two explained how your skin's health does not stop at the superficial level but is affected by the internal workings of your body, hormones, digestion, any allergies and intolerances, lack of or too much exercise, and the accumulation of choices about how you live your life.

If you have a specific skin condition such as acne or rosacea or have noticed that your skin is prematurely ageing, either from hormonal imbalances or sun damage, the next section will help you determine what type of acne/rosacea/skin condition you have. It will also provide a greater understanding of how you can help yourself.

There is information on what vitamins to look for in your skin products to help your skin heal. I have also given you a treatment programme using my skin care products, which I know will support your skin's health while you are dealing with the internal factors. Remember, your skin condition may be quite complex and a symptom of a deeper problem; therefore, you may require the support of a qualified natural therapist for further testing and support. To help you understand the complex nature of your skin and how your health affects your skin, see the summary in Figure 9.

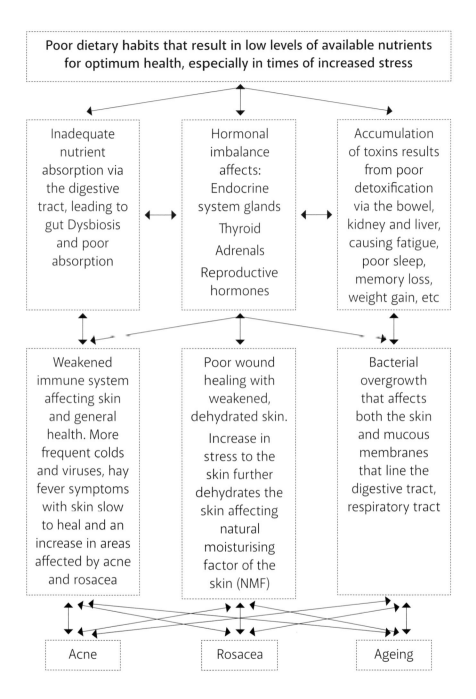

Poor dietary habits that result in low levels of available nutrients for optimum health, especially in times of increased stress

Inadequate nutrient absorption via the digestive tract, leading to gut Dysbiosis and poor absorption

Hormonal imbalance affects:
Endocrine system glands
Thyroid
Adrenals
Reproductive hormones

Accumulation of toxins results from poor detoxification via the bowel, kidney and liver, causing fatigue, poor sleep, memory loss, weight gain, etc

Weakened immune system affecting skin and general health. More frequent colds and viruses, hay fever symptoms with skin slow to heal and an increase in areas affected by acne and rosacea

Poor wound healing with weakened, dehydrated skin.
Increase in stress to the skin further dehydrates the skin affecting natural moisturising factor of the skin (NMF)

Bacterial overgrowth that affects both the skin and mucous membranes that line the digestive tract, respiratory tract

Acne

Rosacea

Ageing

ACNE

❧

W hether you suffer from teenage acne with constant pimples and zits to mature acne, the results on your health and self-esteem are the same and very debilitating, in my experience. There are three general types of acne; however, some can be medication-driven alone and reflective of poor nutrient levels. To get the most out of this section, it is important that you are as objective as possible so that you can identify the underlying issues. Complete the questionnaires, observe and chart your morning temperatures and be aware of hormonal imbalances when you experience skin changes in your cycle.

If you don't need to use the contraceptive pill for contraception, consider stopping it so that your hormones can return to balance and, once your type is identified, go through the lifestyle overhaul. Most importantly, give yourself time to heal and return to balance. In most instances it will take up to three months to see consistent change and stabilisation.

So what is acne?

Acne is the name given to a skin condition where your sebaceous gland, situated in your dermis, is constantly overstimulated to make more oil/lipids this is usually through hormonal changes, food allergies/intolerances and your metabolism. It starts when greasy secretions from the skin's sebaceous glands (oil glands) plug the tiny openings for hair follicles (plugged pores). If the openings are large, the clogs take the form of blackheads: small, flat spots with dark centres. If the openings stay small, the clogs take the form of whiteheads: small, flesh-coloured bumps. Both types of plugged pores can develop into swollen, tender inflammations or pimples, or deeper lumps or nodules. Depending on what skin products you are using they can strip the protective barrier of your skin that fights bacteria, leaving your skin more susceptible to an overgrowth of bacteria, thus infection and further inflammation occur. Your skin can them become more stressed and struggle to heal itself if there are nutritional deficiencies and so the cycle of acne begins. Nodules associated with severe cases of acne (cystic acne) are firm swellings below the skin's surface that become inflamed, tender and sometimes infected.

Acne lesions are most common on the face, but they can also occur on the neck, chest, back, shoulders and upper arms.

TYPES OF ACNE PIMPLES

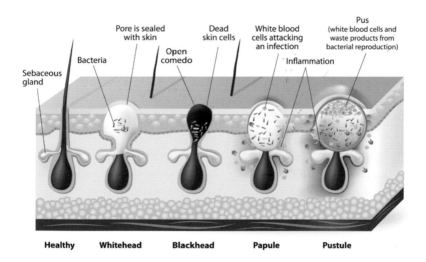

Figure 9: Types of acne pimples

> **Clinical note:**
> I find this is more significant when your iodine and vitamin D levels are low.

Most acne can fit into three types *(see below)*. In my experience, whilst antibiotics and Roaccutane (Roaccutane is a medication that is used to treat acne by drying the sebacaeous gland's fluid therefore reducing swelling. Fortunately it may also affect lots of other glands and membranes of your body) may treat the symptoms initially, it doesn't treat the problem and why you have acne. Being an acne sufferer myself for over 30 years, I wanted to understand the problem rather than continue to suffer the long-term side effects of synthetic drugs, antibiotics and harsh skin products. I was sick of being told "It's only acne!" To me, it was a debilitating condition that took away my self-confidence and robbed me of my right to feel beautiful.

Through this journey I have discovered that your skin is a mirror of what is happening in your body and the imbalances, deficiencies and disharmony. The next section is very exciting as it gives you all the information you ever needed to know about how to have acne-free skin.

Type 1 acne

Digestive imbalance — *Candida/insulin resistance*

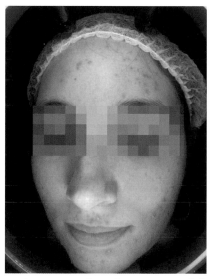

Figure 10: Type 1 acne
Photo used with permission from
LSM Clinic client library

Most people that fit into this category may experience breakouts often, infrequently or monthly. They typically appear on the upper cheeks, temples or forehead. Severe cases can spread onto other parts of the face and/ or body. In my clinical experience, they will be worse when your levels of vitamin D, iodine and zinc are low as well as if your diet is dominated with processed foods, such as two-minute noodles, pizza, sandwiches, dairy-containing products and high-sugar drinks, including fruit juices with concentrated fructose. To start the process of reclaiming your skin and your health, revise the foods that you eat on a daily basis and include your comfort foods such as chocolate, bread and ice cream — often they are your undoing. If you are unsure of where to start, the food programme will give you some ideas and the recipes are also a helpful starting point. You can build on them after you gain more confidence. Replace cow's milk with nut milk and cheese with Vegusto cheese if you feel you can't go without cheese. My clients who regularly swim in a chlorinated pool find this regular exposure to chlorine has the ability to affect their thyroid gland by blocking the gland's ability to function normally and receive its hormones that signal it to function. If this is affecting you it will affect your metabolism of the food and drinks that you ingest as well as your energy levels, hormone production and effectiveness of existing hormones and sleep patterns. *(For more information, see "Your skin and your hormonal health: the complex connection" on page 30-49.)*

Use of long-term antibiotics causes digestive disruption and destroys the delicate balance of good and bad bacteria; therefore, kefir and probiotic support are essential on a daily basis. Daily exercise is vital to reduce insulin resistance *(see the insulin resistance questionnaire to check if you may be affected on page 93)*. If you have been on medication specifically designed to treat acne, be aware that rehydrating the skin, both your dermis and your epidermis, to improve its health and resistance is vital because most acne medications are aimed at drying up the sebaceous gland's oil production, which is normally designed to maintain your skin's hydration and resilience to dehydration. In my experience clinically, I have found that your skin care should start with using topically B3 concentrate and a hydrating formula that consists of vitamins such as L-hyaluronic acid, allantoin L-mandelic and L-ascorbic acid, which is vitamin C. *(See Table 3 on page 52.)*

Type 2 acne (PCOS/insulin resistance)

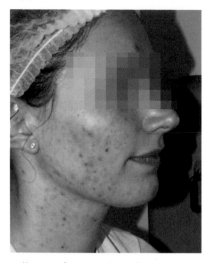

Figure 11: Type 2 acne
Photo used with permission from LSM Clinic client library

If you have type 2 acne, you will have oily skin as your sebaceous glands overproduce sebum. This stimulus is from internal triggers such as: diet (insulin-like growth factor — IGF — from dairy products); sluggish metabolism (possibly low iodine levels); and low thyroid health and hormonal imbalance (from the contraceptive pill or for males from body building products and hormonal stimulants that you buy online). The breakouts are in the "male beard line" area. Other factors that result in this type of acne are early or late-stage PCOS (polycystic ovarian syndrome) and/or insulin resistance. *(Check the insulin resistance questionnaire on page 100 to see if this is relevant to you.)*

I have seen severe cases can spread on the face and/or to the body. Some thin teenage males may have a testosterone imbalance if their cystic acne is on the beard line or high oestrogen levels that can result from xenoestrogens *(see Table 4 on page 54)*. Other clues for type 2 are an increase in facial hair, painful menstruation, low vitamin D levels, low iodine and low energy. This may indicate not only a hormonal imbalance, but also a food intolerance and/or allergy, which is why it is important to keep a diary.

Clinical note: A steroid cycle resulting in type 2 acne.

A young man came to me struggling with wounds from type 2 acne. They were worse on his chest and stomach but he also had them on his back and arms to a lesser degree. At the time he was a keen body builder who started using steroids, namely testosterone enanthate.

He stated to me that, "During the cycle [using the hormone] my diet was extremely clean with home-cooked meals and I really didn't need to use other supplements because ... well steroids just blow them all out of the water."

After trying antibiotics and other treaments, his acne had developed into wounds and was not improving. Figure 13 shows his skin at first diagnosis. Figure 14 is taken four months later after treatment. We had discovered that he was using testosterone-stimulating powders, he was intolerant to dairy, he was also low in iodine, zinc, vitamins A and D and his adrenal glands were exhausted from being overstimulated by the steroids. Once these problems were corrected we were able to heal his skin and he was able to hug his wife without pain!

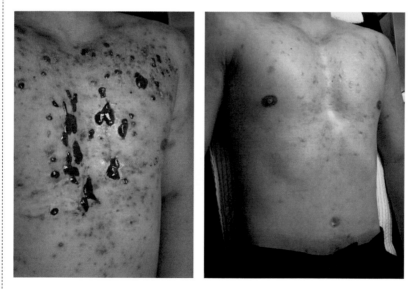

Figure 12: **Client with burnt out hormones and low iodine, vitamin D and poor digestive health from body building products purchased online and lifestyle.** Photo used with permission from LSM Clinic client library

Figure 13: **Treatment results after four months.** Photo used with permission from LSM Clinic client library.

Unique points about type 2 acne

As with type 1 acne, it is imperative that you change your food choices initially as a significant part of type 2 acne results from poor sugar (insulin resistance) and fructose metabolism as well as inadequate oestrogen metabolism from low fiber intake as well as low iodine levels. I would advise excluding fruit from your diet in the short-term, that is, for approximately one month, including all natural fruit until the skin recovers to reduce the level of insulin resistance. One of the best indications will be that your skin is not breaking out as much and healing faster if you do get a breakout.

Type 3 acne

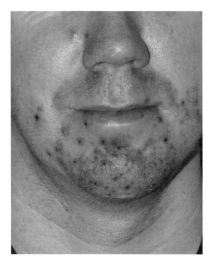

Figure 14: Type 3 acne
Photo used with permission from LSM Clinic client library

Type 3 acne tends to be a more episodic form of acne but can also transition into type 1 or type 2. It may be triggered by:

• diet

• stress overload, resulting in hormonal imbalance

• exposure to toxins, not only in food but also personal care products

• skin product irritants

• external stressors, such as flying

• physical stressors, such as an episode of antibiotics and other medications such as steroids, inhalers and so on, that changes your digestive health.

It is often described as "occasional breakouts". However, I have found that type 3 may also be related to nutritional insufficiencies from a stressful event such as a short illness, car accident or anaesthetic that results in low levels of iodine, vitamin D or zinc. Your body needs more nutrients when it is under stressful situations such as those listed above. Other stressful events can include exams, a first date, lack of sleep, the start of a new job, relationship or family changes, a death in the family, and so on. Your skin may be worse in winter than it is in summer due to lack of sun exposure.

Medications may also be a trigger for type 3 acne; such as the use of the contraceptive pill, antidepressants, antacids, but also medications you may not think of such as steroid medications, including topical for problems such as dermatitis and eczema, and the use of inhalers that change the flora of the mouth. Note that oil pulling is a great way to regain a healthy mouth and digestive system and counteract some of these triggers *(see the section on oil pulling on page 76).*

Clinical case:

Claire was a university student studying the arts. She was very focused on her course and glad that it was coming to an end. I saw her after she had a breakout of acne that did not clear up as it had done previously. As we discussed her history she told me that she got the occasional pimple and it was always worse just before her period and when she pulled an "all nighter" to finish a paper. She had been on a course of Roaccutane in her early 20s but didn't like how it made her feel and she suffered blood noses and a dry mouth as a result of it so she didn't want to do that again.

In the previous nine months, she had had the flu really badly and been in bed for a week. After that, her skin just did not seem to heal and she had embarrassing, large pimples all the time.

This is not an uncommon story as the body is under a constant amount of stress when you are at university, working shift work, or in a stressful job such as in the emergency services and so on. It only took one or two more demanding incidents to tip Claire over the edge of her optimal health.

On testing, Claire was low in vitamin D and iodine and this was affecting her thyroid and general metabolic health. She was not taking the contraceptive pill so that was not a factor.

On changing the food that she eats, eliminating allergens and making better choices with managing timetables and the stress of day-to-day demands, Claire's skin returned to health over the next four months.

Now, with good skin care and replacing the deficit in nutrients, Claire has no breakouts and manages her stress levels much better. She is also mindful that she needs to plan her meals so she doesn't get caught out.

Lifestyle overhaul for acne

1. **Define** which **type of acne** you have.

2. **Treat your skin with nutrient-dense topical skin care products** that feed and nurture, reduce redness and congestion, remodel and heal your skin within your renewal cycle. Remember, depending on your age, your skin renews itself every 30–60 days. *(See Table 11 on page 187 if you are interested in our skin care products.)*

3. **Improve your digestive function** by eliminating processed foods and sugary drinks including energy and sports drinks - Complete your food diary to assess for dysbosis, allergies or intolerances. Add fiber daily with food from table 3 page 52. Increase your daily filtered water intake, especially on waking and before bed. Eliminate dairy — your calcium levels can be managed with greens and nuts, such as almonds. Ensure you have high-protein foods daily to assist skin healing — it is very important for vegetarians to find a good protein source that is not dairy-based. Remove allergens and intolerances and start changing your habits.

4. **Correct any hormonal or metabolic imbalance** — assess your thyroid health using the basal metabolic temperature method. Remove harmful chemicals and petrochemicals that are known hormone disruptors from your personal care products, cleaning agents and household items. Buy organic or spray-free food whenever you can at the farmers' markets, since they are a great place to get good-quality food at a reasonable price. Check your oestrogen status for oestrogen dominance. Remember, you will need to increase your non-carbohydrate fibre intake if you are positive. Check your vitamin D status and include the **Heal & Reveal** skin product as an essential part of your skin rehabilitation programme if you are using our products and your vitamin D is low.

5. **Evaluate the effectiveness of your sleep, exercise patterns and exposure to stress** and make the necessary changes. If you are breaking out after exercise you may be iodine deficient.

6. **You may need further testing** such as vitamin D levels, thyroid function or a salivary hormonal test for stress and/or reproductive

hormones. Seek the assistance of a natural health practitioner to assist and guide you.

Acne checklist

✓ Use skin care that feeds your skin — feed, remodel and heal your skin *(as described in Table 12 if you wish to try our products).*

✓ Improve your digestive function by eliminating processed foods and sugary drinks — complete your food diary to assess for dysbosis, allergies or intolerances. Add fiber daily with food from *Table 3: Nutrients and their functions for good health page 52.*

✓ Start a probiotic morning and night if you are taking any medications or have dysbosis

✓ Increase your daily filtered water intake, especially on waking and before bed.

✓ Eliminate dairy — your calcium levels can be managed with greens and nuts such as almonds.

✓ Ensure you have high-protein foods daily to help support skin health and healing.

✓ Start a good quality vitamin D supplement until you know what your levels are. You can then adjust as you may need a high dose of vitamin D to start with if your results are low.

✓ Reassess your sleep, exercise patterns and stress — see where you can make changes and improvements, remembering that your skin health is the accumulation of your choices and habits to date.

✓ Eliminate toxins from your hair care, toothpaste, make-up and so on *(see "Chemicals to avoid" on page 57).*

✓ Do a treatment mask at least weekly but do not use harsh exfoliates or mechanical abrasives.

✓ Commence oil pulling daily for 15–20 minutes — be aware that you may have some subtle detoxification reactions to this regime.

✓ Increase non-carbohydrate fibre intake with meal plan changes on a daily basis. *(See our website www.marianrubock.com.au under "Your wellness" for links to our recommendations.)*

✓ Check your basal metabolic temperature for any possible thyroid implications and continue to monitor if you are taking extra iodine due to a low result.

✓ Complete your diary, noting, if female, when your menstrual cycle falls and any skin changes after eating.

✓ Enjoy chemical-free and, where possible, organic foods to reduce your exposure to herbicides and pesticides.

✓ Exercise daily for at least 40 minutes — monitor your steps or distance. Increase your incidental exercise wherever possible. This is especially important if you have type 1 and 2 acne.

✓ You may need further testing such as vitamin D levels, thyroid function, Iodine levels and stress and reproductive hormonal levels. Seek the assistance of a natural health practitioner to assist and guide you and get you on the right dosages.

Important clinical note for skin product use:

If you wish to try our products, please refer to Table 12. Start with the **basic trio** and then add **Heal & Reveal** if you are low on vitamin D.

Once your skin is healing, you can add the **Skin Renewal Stimulator** to further reduce inflammation, infection, blocked pores and promote healing.

If you feel you need exfoliation, the **Skin Glo** is a great product that exfoliates without the harsh scratching and damage to your skin.

Once your skin is stable, add **Naturally A Starter** and work your way up to Full Strength to heal the scarring, and thicken and tighten the skin. The Naturally A products are also great to control the amount of sebum your skin secretes.

Our skin care products are concentrated so excess use *is not better, just wasteful.* There is also a great spot treatment you can use, **Heal & Vanish,** but, again, please remember a small amount is only what is needed on clean skin.

Table 12: LSM skin care products for acne

LSM skin care products	Acne protocol How to use	Type 1 acne	Type 2 acne	Type 3 acne
Start with basic trio				
Gentle Cleanse	Apply 1–2 pumps to damp skin and lather. Rinse thoroughly. Use morning and evening.	✓		✓
Deep Cleanse			✓	
Serum B3	1 pump.	✓	✓	✓
Balance & Hydrate	1–2 pumps.	✓ Apply am & pm.	✓	✓
Extra support once stable on basic trio				
Heal & Reveal	Spray onto skin morning and night. May mix with Serum B3.	✓	✓	✓
Revive & Restore	May need to use instead of Balance and Hydrate if recently been on Roaccutane.	✓	✓	✓
Skin Renewal Stimulator	May use with Serum B3 after 2 weeks of using vitamin D serum and then only at night for a month. Please be aware that you may experience some tingling, which is normal. Once your skin has got used to the product you may use it morning and night.	✓	✓	✓
Heal and Vanish Spot Treatment	Apply to pimples on clean skin as desired.	✓ Use sparingly on spot.	✓ Use sparingly on spot.	✓ Use sparingly on spot.
Skin Glo — fruit-based exfoliant	Place on clean skin and leave for 15–30 minutes. Rinse fully and apply nourishing serums.	✓ Apply weekly.	✓ Apply weekly.	✓ Apply weekly.
Reverse scarring, rebuild and stabilise				
Naturally A Starter		✓	✓	✓

LSM skin care products	Acne protocol How to use	Type 1 acne	Type 2 acne	Type 3 acne
Naturally A Mid Strength	May advance to Mid Strength after using at least two bottles of Starter.	Apply morning and night.	Apply morning and night.	Apply morning and night.
Naturally A Full Strength	May advance to Full Strength after using at least two bottles of Mid Strength.	Apply morning and night.	Apply morning and night.	Apply morning and night.
Eye care				
Rejuvenating Eye Serum	May use either eye serums or both and alternate between morning and night application.	✓	✓	✓
Eye Nurture		✓	✓	✓
Sun protection				
Sun Defend No Tint	Non-greasy, non-comedogenic formula.	✓	✓	✓
Sun Defend Tinted Light/Medium/dark	Non-greasy, non-comedogenic formula.	✓	✓	✓

ROSACEA

☙

Rosacea is an interesting skin problem to treat. In my experience, my clients have one thing in common, other than persistent redness and irritation: they over-think! This puts a lot of pressure on your mental and emotional stress response and affects the skin as it is uniquely tied to the nervous and digestive system *(see "Your skin and your hormonal health: the complex connection" on page 30-49).*

Acne medications and oral antibiotics may sometimes be prescribed for rosacea. However, their long-term use comes with complications for other organs such as your liver and further skin dehydration as they stop the sebaceous glands from producing sebum, which supports skin hydration. Topical antibiotics may give short-term relief for localised inflammation and congestion, but unfortunately do not treat the cause. Clients who have had rosacea in their 30s and 40s suffer more symptoms as they go through andropause and menopause. This is due to the hormonal connection of rosacea to your metabolism which affects your digestive enzymes and the amount of hydrochloric acid you secrete. If you are low in iodine this symptom will be amplified.

Because your body and skin do not operate independently, the health of your body's other systems will affect the health of your skin. Prescription medications, over-the-counter pain medications such as HRT, the contraceptive pill, inhalers, antacids and codeine-based pain relief can affect and change the receptors in your digestive and endocrine system and reduce its ability to maintain balance, therefore creating more digestive inflammation and metabolic imbalance. So, where possible, use these medications with caution. Medications may sometimes work, depending on your type of rosacea, but they do not treat the cause.

As we discuss the types of rosacea and the treatment recommendations we are talking about dealing with the underlying causes so that we can calm and heal your skin. Please be patient with yourself as you go through this process as it takes time for your body to heal. There will be ups and downs along the way as your body starts on its journey to rebalance and heal.

Type 1 rosacea

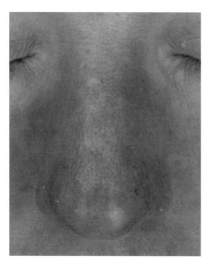

Figure 15: Type 1 rosacea
Photo used with permission from
LSM Clinic client library

Most people with type 1 rosacea experience the following symptoms:

- Redness and itching on the tip of your nose.
- Persistent flushing.
- Redness and sensitivity.
- Dry skin that may burn or sting.

This form of rosacea usually occurs from inflammation of the upper digestive tract or throat, such as chronic mild gastritis, or allergies localised to the nasal passages and back of the throat. It may also be caused by overconsumption of alcohol and/or smoking. Further causes are stress, low iodine levels, because iodine acts as a natural antiseptic in our stomach, and resulting hormonal imbalance.

Clinical note

Some clients with iodine deficiency are now improving faster with the correct dose of iodine, which is essential for supporting the secretion of hydrochloric acid. It acts as a stomach antiseptic for bacteria, fungi, virus and other harmful microorganisms and detoxifies chemicals in the body, just to name a few of its functions. If you have rosacea, you should consider undergoing the iodine challenge test (see "Are you lacking iodine?" on page 43).

Type 2 rosacea

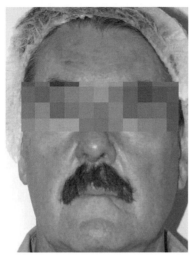

Figure 16: Type 2 rosacea
Photo used with permission from
LSM Clinic client library

If you have type 2 rosacea you may experience the following symptoms:

- Flushing, redness, sensitivity or dry skin that may burn or sting on the sides of your nose.
- Small bumps and pimples or acne-like breakouts and/or if your skin gets coarser and thicker, with a bumpy texture.

This form of rosacea usually results from digestive inflammation around the stomach and or lung inflammation with a history of using inhalants such as Ventolin and allergies. It is most likely related to acid reflux, *H. Pylori,* ulcers, gastritis or the body's ability to ward off viruses, bacteria, fungi and other microorganism as is the case when you are iodine deficient. Lifestyle stresses, food allergies and hormonal menopause/andropause are also factors.

Type 3 rosacea

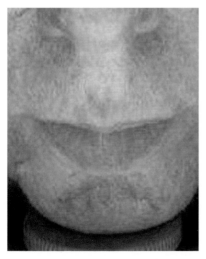

Figure 17: Type 3 rosacea
Photo used with permission from
LSM Clinic client library

If you have type 3 rosacea, you may experience lower digestive inflammation, causing symptoms such as:

- Persistent flushing on your cheeks, temples, forehead and/or eyes.
- Flushing, redness, sensitivity or dry skin that may burn or sting.
- Small bumps and pimples or acne-like breakouts and/or if your skin gets coarser and thicker, with a bumpy texture.

This form of rosacea typically results from inflammation to the large and small intestine. The most common causes include Candidiasis, gluten/gliadin sensitivity, allergies or chronic conditions such as irritable bowel syndrome and nutritional deficiencies such as iodine that prevent your body from restoring balance and maintaining a strong immune system *(see Table 3 on page 52)*. It may also be the result of insulin resistance and a breakdown in your body's natural defences, causing immune stress and hormonal imbalance.

Lifestyle overhaul for rosacea

1. **Define** which **type of rosacea** you have.

2. **Treat the skin with nutrient-dense skin care products** — remember your skin, hair and nails are the last structures and organs to get nutrients so it is important, for the skin's recovery, to apply topical, nutritionally supportive skin care products. Also, please be patient with your skin as you are working within your skin's renewal cycle. Depending on your age, your skin renews itself every 30–60 days. *(Using the LSM skin care plan, start with the **basic trio** and add **Heal & Reveal** if your vitamin D levels are low.)*

3. **Improve your digestive function** by eliminating processed foods and sugary drinks and concentrated juices drinks. Complete your food diary to assess for any food allergies or intolerances and look for bloating, fatigue or fogginess an hour after meals as well changes in bowel habits and cravings. Increase your daily filtered water intake, especially on waking and before bed. Eliminate dairy — your calcium levels can be managed with greens and nuts such as almonds. Start oil pulling daily; it is great for balancing your digestive tract and therefore is very effective for rosacea, as it is for all skin conditions. Check for digestive disorders such as dysbosis and start probiotic therapy.

   Ensure you have high-protein foods daily to help support skin health and healing. Start a vitamin D supplement until you know what your levels are. You can then adjust as you may need a high dose of vitamin D to start with if your results are low. Increase non-carbohydrate fibre intake with meal plan changes on a daily basis. *(See our website for links in the section "Your Wellness".)*

4. **Evaluate the effectiveness of your sleep, exercise patterns and exposure to stress.** See where you can make changes and improvements, remembering that your skin health is the accumulation of your choices and habits to date. Exercise daily for at least 40 minutes — monitor your steps or distance. Increase your incidental exercise wherever possible. This is especially important if you have type 1 and 2 rosacea.

5. **Correct any hormonal or metabolic imbalance.** Eliminate toxins from your hair care, toothpaste, make-up and so on *(see "Chemicals to avoid" on page 54 and 57)*. Check your basal metabolic temperature for any possible thyroid implications and continue to monitor if you are taking extra iodine due to a low result. Complete your diary, noting, if female, when your menstrual cycle falls and any skin changes. Enjoy chemical-free and, where possible, organic foods to reduce your exposure to herbicides and pesticides.

6. **You may need further testing** such as: thyroid function, iodine, stress and reproductive hormonal levels. Seek the assistance of a natural health practitioner to assist and guide you.

Rosacea checklist

✓ Start skin care that feeds your skin — feed, remodel and heal your skin *(as described in Table 13 on page 195, if you wish to use our products)*.

✓ Improve your digestive function by eliminating processed foods and sugary drinks — complete your food diary to assess for dysbosis, allergies or intolerances. Add fiber daily with food from *Table 3: Nutrients and their functions for good health, page 52.*

✓ Increase your daily filtered water intake, especially on waking and before bed.

✓ Eliminate dairy — your calcium levels can be managed with greens and nuts such as almonds.

✓ Ensure you have high-protein foods daily to help support skin health and healing.

✓ Start a vitamin D supplement until you establish what your levels are. You can work with a health professional to adjust this.

- ✓ Reassess your sleep, exercise patterns and stress — see where you can make changes and improvements, remembering that your skin health is the accumulation of your choices and habits to date.

- ✓ Eliminate toxins from your hair care, toothpaste, make-up and so on *(see "Chemicals to avoid" on page 57).*

- ✓ Commence oil pulling daily for 15–20 minutes — be aware that you may have some subtle detoxification reactions. *(See section on oil pulling on page 76)*

- ✓ Increase your fibre intake with meal plan changes on a daily basis.

- ✓ Check your basal metabolic temperature for any possible thyroid implications and continue to monitor if you are taking extra Iodine due to a low result as you want to see your temperature improve and increase to 36.5° Celsius or 97.7° Fahrenheit. (Work with a natural practitioner on this one area.)

- ✓ Complete your diary, note events such as, if female, when your menstrual cycle falls and any skin changes after eating, reflux and tiredness after meals. Are there foods that make your sleeping worse or make you snore?

- ✓ Exercise daily for at least 40 minutes — monitor your steps or distance. Increase your incidental exercise wherever possible. Note if you are tired an hour after exercise or the next day.

- ✓ You will need further testing such as vitamin D levels, thyroid function, iodine levels and stress and reproductive hormonal levels. Seek the assistance of a natural health practitioner to assist and guide you.

Important clinical note for skin product use: If you wish to try our products, please refer to Table 13 on page 195. Start with the **basic trio** and then add **Heal & Reveal** if you are low on vitamin D.

Once your skin is healing, you can add the ***Skin renewal stimulator*** to further reduce inflammation, and promote healing and skin thickening. Use it only at night to start with and be aware it may produce a tingling sensation for some people.

If you feel you need exfoliation, ***Skin Glo*** is a great product that exfoliates without harsh scratching and damage to your skin.

Once your skin is stable, add **Naturally A Starter** and work your way up to Full Strength to reverse the damage, ageing and thinning of the skin. The Naturally A products are also great to thicken the skin and improve your skin's health.

More of your product is not better. Please use only as we have recommended so you don't waste your skin care products.

Table 13: LSM skin care products for rosacea

LSM skin care products	Rosacea protocol How to use	Type 1	Type 2	Type 3
Start with basic trio				
Gentle Cleanse	Apply 1–2 pumps to damp skin and lather. Rinse thoroughly. Use morning and evening.	✓	✓	✓
Vitamin B3 Serum	1 pump.	✓	✓	✓
Balance & Hydrate	1–2 pumps.	✓	✓	✓
Extra support once stable on basic trio				
Heal & Reveal	Mix 1–2 sprays with B3 Serum.	✓	✓	✓
Revive & Restore — for severely dehydrated skin instead of Balance & Hydrate	Rehydration.	✓	✓	✓
Skin Renewal Stimulator	May use with Serum B3 after 2 weeks of using vitamin D serum and then only at night for a month. Please be aware that you may experience some tingling, which is normal. Once your skin has got used to the product you may use it morning and night.	✓	✓	✓
Skin Glo	Place on clean skin and leave for 10–20 minutes. Rinse fully and use vitamin B3 and Balance & Hydrate.	✓ Apply weekly.	✓ Apply weekly.	✓ Apply weekly.

LSM skin care products	Rosacea protocol How to use	Type 1	Type 2	Type 3
Reverse damage ageing and thicken skin				
Naturally A Starter	Start rebuilding and advance to stronger vitamin A as skin improves. Only advance if the skin does not feel dry.	✓ Apply night only to start then add morning dose.	✓ Apply night only to start then add morning dose.	✓ Apply night only to start then add morning dose.
Naturally A Mid Strength	May advance to Mid Strength after using at least two bottles of Starter.	✓ May use morning and night.	✓ May use morning and night.	✓ May use morning and night.
Naturally A Full Strength	May advance to Full Strength after using at least two bottles of Mid Strength.	✓ May use morning and night.	✓ May use morning and night.	✓ May use morning and night.
Eye care				
Rejuvenating Eye Serum	May use either eye serums or both and alternate between morning and night application.	✓	✓	✓
Eye Nurture		✓ Apply 1 pump morning and night	✓ Apply 1 pump morning and night	✓ Apply 1 pump morning and night
Sun protection				
Sun Defend Tinted Light/Medium	Nourishing anti-radiation formula to protect against the sun.	✓ Apply daily, best 20 minutes prior to sun exposure.	✓ Apply daily, best 20 minutes prior to sun exposure.	✓ Apply daily, best 20 minutes prior to sun exposure.
Sun defend No Tint	Nourishing anti-radiation formula to protect against the sun.	✓ Apply daily, best 20 minutes prior to sun exposure.	✓ Apply daily, best 20 minutes prior to sun exposure.	✓ Apply daily, best 20 minutes prior to sun exposure.

Remember, you need to add changes to your diet and lifestyle as well and check for hormonal imbalance such as oestrogen dominance, insulin resistance, low thyroid function, low iodine levels and stress hormone imbalance. Writing everything down will help you understand where your body needs support and see patterns of how your skin responds to certain situations and foods.

AGEING AND HEALTHY SKIN

ॐ

You can't avoid getting chronologically older, but you can take steps to keep your skin looking youthful and healthy. Premature ageing occurs with the onset of perimenopause, sun damage and nutritional insufficiencies, as you can see in Figure 18. When you correct these imbalances and deficiencies, you have the opportunity to not only turn back the hands of time visually but internally. This, in turn, provides support for life's ups and downs and a reduction in the inflammation that occurs so much more easily as we get older. With a few simple lifestyle changes and a good-quality skin care regime, you are on the right path.

Clinical note:

I have worked with many clients who have wanted to turn back the hands of time and feel better about themselves. Sometimes it is a wedding that is the trigger for them coming to see me; other times it's a change in their lifestyle and relationship status. I remember one lovely lady who sat in front of me and asked, "Can you make me visible again?"

I asked what she meant by this comment and she said that too often she would be standing at a retail counter and would be ignored. Just trying to get served was a nightmare. She was always overlooked for someone else who was, in her eyes, younger, prettier, more youthful.

As we started talking, she told me that her motivation for life was low; she was lacking in energy and felt every day was a struggle. She disliked learning new things and felt overwhelmed at social events, so tended to avoid them. This was a problem for her partner, who was very social and enjoyed having her by his side. She said he would tease and say, "Come on, you grumpy old thing!"

I could see this was an intelligent woman going through menopause, which, to date, had been a nightmare.

We discussed her issues and put together a plan to fix them, as well as addressing how she felt about herself and her skin. This included balancing her hormones and thyroid, using skin care and regularly doing treatments to reverse the signs of ageing.

Five months later, when I asked her how she was, she beamed at me and said, "I am not invisible any more!" She proceeded to tell me the story of her experience when she last went shopping, being at a shopping counter and how it felt to be seen. I suspect that as her confidence, energy and tolerance had grown as much as her skin health had changed which resulted in her feeling better about herself and everyone around her responded to this. It is at these times when I love what I do the most. The look on my client's face was precious and I felt very grateful that I had been part of her transformation.

Ageing comes in many forms, some of which you may not expect to age your skin; whilst others you will be familiar with, such as:

- Sun damage.
- Body inflammation.
- Hormonal imbalance and decreasing levels of hormones.
- Lack of nutrition-dense food or absorption and/or both due to low levels of beneficial microbiome.
- Dehydration.
- Lack of regular exercise.
- Increased levels of uncontrolled stress, affecting lifestyle and sleep.
- Lack of good-quality sleep.
- Hypothyroidism.
- Low levels of vital nutrients such as vitamins A and D, zinc, magnesium and iodine, just to name a few.

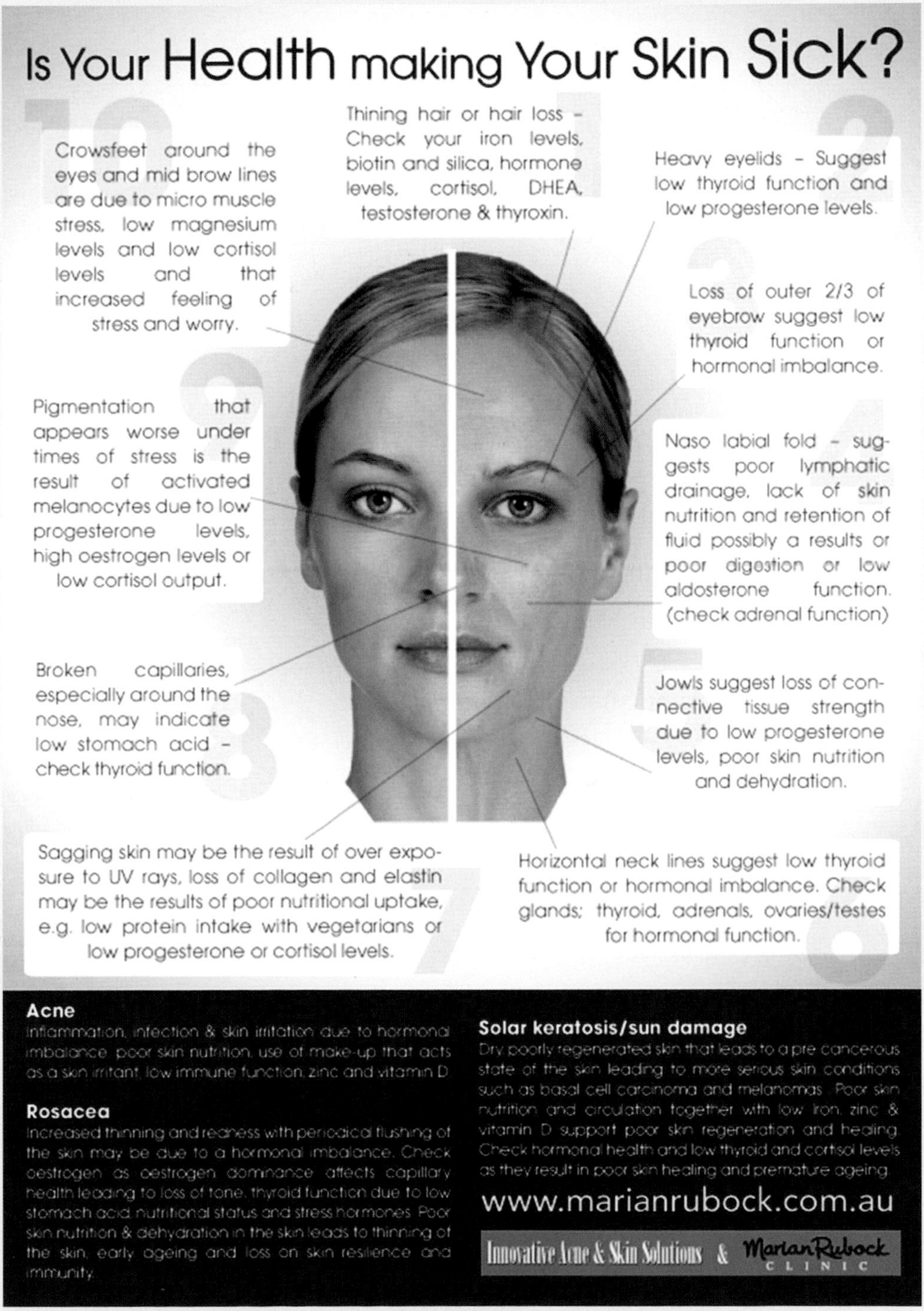

Is Your Health making Your Skin Sick?

Crowsfeet around the eyes and mid brow lines are due to micro muscle stress, low magnesium levels and low cortisol levels and that increased feeling of stress and worry.

Thining hair or hair loss – Check your iron levels, biotin and silica, hormone levels, cortisol, DHEA, testosterone & thyroxin.

Heavy eyelids – Suggest low thyroid function and low progesterone levels.

Loss of outer 2/3 of eyebrow suggest low thyroid function or hormonal imbalance.

Pigmentation that appears worse under times of stress is the result of activated melanocytes due to low progesterone levels, high oestrogen levels or low cortisol output.

Naso labial fold – suggests poor lymphatic drainage, lack of skin nutrition and retention of fluid possibly a results or poor digestion or low aldosterone function. (check adrenal function)

Broken capillaries, especially around the nose, may indicate low stomach acid – check thyroid function.

Jowls suggest loss of connective tissue strength due to low progesterone levels, poor skin nutrition and dehydration.

Sagging skin may be the result of over exposure to UV rays, loss of collagen and elastin may be the results of poor nutritional uptake, e.g. low protein intake with vegetarians or low progesterone or cortisol levels.

Horizontal neck lines suggest low thyroid function or hormonal imbalance. Check glands; thyroid, adrenals, ovaries/testes for hormonal function.

Acne
Inflammation, infection & skin irritation due to hormonal imbalance poor skin nutrition, use of make-up that acts as a skin irritant, low immune function, zinc and vitamin D

Rosacea
Increased thinning and redness with periodical flushing of the skin may be due to a hormonal imbalance. Check oestrogen as oestrogen dominance affects capillary health leading to loss of tone, thyroid function due to low stomach acid, nutritional status and stress hormones. Poor skin nutrition & dehydration in the skin leads to thinning of the skin, early ageing and loss on skin resilience and immunity.

Solar keratosis/sun damage
Dry, poorly regenerated skin that leads to a pre cancerous state of the skin leading to more serious skin conditions such as basal cell carcinoma and melanomas. Poor skin nutrition and circulation together with low iron, zinc & vitamin D support poor skin regeneration and healing. Check hormonal health and low thyroid and cortisol levels as they result in poor skin healing and premature ageing.

www.marianrubock.com.au

Innovative Acne & Skin Solutions & *Marian Rubock* CLINIC

Figure 18: Is your health making your skin sick?

When you use chirally correct skin care, with vitamins, peptides and hydration, your skin will regenerate and rejuvenate, resulting in a more youthful and hydrated complexion, with fewer lines and wrinkles. Since your skin, nails and hair are the last organ and structures to receive nutrients, it makes good sense to feed your skin.

The best way to give your skin back its youthful glow is by feeding it with natural materials, rebuilding it from the inside out, thus helping to activate its own healing processes. While chemicals and surgical procedures, such as Botox, synthetic fillers and facelifts can provide a temporary solution, they don't address any of the underlying factors that are contributing to your ageing.

Fresh, healthy-looking skin is firm, plump, moist, elastic and supple. Maintaining skin health is a complex task for your body as your skin mirrors healthy immune, digestive and hormonal systems. Together with good-quality food, restful sleep, regular exercise, a reduction in toxic exposures and filtered water for hydration, these factors will help you turn back the hands of time.

Lifestyle overhaul for anti-ageing

1. **Treat your skin with chirally correct skin care products.** Remember your skin, hair and nails are the last organ and structures to get nutrients, so it is important, for the skin's recovery, that you apply nutritionally supportive skin care. Also, please be patient with your skin as you are working within the renewal cycle. Depending on your age, your skin renews itself every 30–60 days. *(Aged 40 years or more, this will be every 60 days.)*

2. **Improve your digestive function** by reducing the amount of processed foods and sugary drinks and alcohol you consume. Increase your daily filtered water intake, especially on waking and before bed. Eliminate dairy — your calcium levels can be managed with greens and nuts, such as almonds. Ensure you have high-protein foods daily, remove allergens, intolerances and start changing your habits. Keep a food diary to support rebuilding and healing with healthy changes. Start oil pulling daily; it is great for improving elimination and the health of your digestive tract and therefore a great anti-ageing strategy.

3. **Correct any hormonal or metabolic imbalance.** Assess your thyroid health using the basal metabolic temperature method. If it is low, have a thyroid check, and remove harmful chemicals and petrochemicals that are known hormone disruptors from your personal care products, cleaning agents and household items. Check your oestrogen status for oestrogen dominance. If you are positive, consider completing a hormone assessment salivary test. If you have completed the Iodine questionnaire and you are over eight points, consider getting your Iodine clearance test done so that you know your level of nutritional deficit and the best dose of iodine to get you back to health.

4. **Evaluate the effectiveness of your sleep, exercise patterns and exposure to stress**. The less stress and inflammation that is in your body, the healthier your skin will be. It is the habits and choices we make every day that have an accumulative benefit, so make yours count!

5. **You may need to do further testing** such as vitamin D levels, thyroid function, or a salivary hormonal check for stress. Seek the assistance of a natural health practitioner to assist and guide you.

Anti-ageing checklist

✓ Start skin care that feeds your skin — feed, remodel and heal your skin *(please refer to Table 14 page 203 if you would like to use our skin care range)*.

✓ Improve your digestive function by eliminating processed foods and sugary and alcoholic drinks — complete your food diary to assess for dysbosis, allergies or intolerances. Add fiber daily with food from *Table 3: Nutrients and their functions for good health page 52*.

✓ Increase your daily filtered water intake, especially on waking and before bed.

✓ Eliminate dairy — your calcium levels can be managed with greens and nuts such as almonds.

✓ Ensure you have high-protein foods daily to help support skin health and general healing in your body.

✓ Start a vitamin D supplement until you know what your levels are. You can work with a health professional to adjust as required.

✓ Reassess your sleep, exercise patterns and stress — see where you can make changes and improvements, remembering that your skin health is the accumulation of your choices and habits to date.

✓ Increase your daily non-carbohydrate-based fibre intake such as inulin or psyllium husks.

✓ Eliminate toxins from your hair care, toothpaste, make-up and so on *(see "Chemicals to avoid", Table 5, on page 57).*

✓ Commence oil pulling daily for 15–20 minutes — be aware that you may have some subtle detoxification reactions.

✓ Check your basal metabolic temperature for any possible thyroid implications and continue to monitor if you are taking extra iodine due to a low result.

✓ Exercise daily for at least 40 minutes — monitor your steps daily for distance, add weight training 3-4 times per week and increase your incidental exercise wherever possible.

✓ You may need further testing such as vitamin D levels, thyroid function, and stress and reproductive hormonal levels if you were positive on any of your questionnaires. Seek the assistance of a natural health practitioner to assist and guide you.

Important clinical note for skin product use: If you wish to try our products, please refer to Table 14. Start with the basic trio and then add **Heal & Reveal** if you are low on vitamin D.

Once your skin is hydrated, you can add the **Skin Renewal Stimulator** to further reduce inflammation, promote skin renewal and skin thickening.

If you feel you need exfoliation the **Skin Glo** is a great product that exfoliates without the harsh scratching and damage to your skin and it really makes your skin Glow!

Once your skin is stable, add **Naturally A Starter** (natural vitamin A) and work your way up to **Full Strength** to reverse the damage, ageing and thinning of the skin. The Naturally A products also feature anti-ageing and skin tightening benefits with the ingredients improving the overall health of your skin.

More of your product is not better. Please use only as we have recommended so you don't waste your skin care products.

Table 14: LSM skin care products for anti-ageing

LSM skin care products	Anti-ageing protocol How to use	When
Start with basic trio		
Deep Cleanse	Apply 1–2 pumps to damp skin and lather. Rinse thoroughly. Use morning and evening. Use Deep Cleanse for a deeper, exfoliating cleanse.	✓ Use morning and night.
Gentle Cleanse		✓ Use morning and night.
B3 Serum	Apply 1 pump and apply to clean skin.	✓ Use morning and night.
Balance and Hydrate	Apply 1-2 pumps on clean skin after B3 serum.	✓ Use morning and night.
Extra support once stable on basic trio		
Skin Renewal Stimulator	Combine with B3 serum at night only. Please be aware that you may experience some tingling, which is normal. Once your skin is used to the product you may use it morning and night.	✓ Great for ageing skin as it resurfaces and removes pigmentation.
Revive & Restore	Apply instead of balance & Hydrate if your skin feels dry or during the winter months.	✓ Use morning and night.
Heal & Reveal Vitamin Serum	You may mix with B3 Serum and Skin Renewal Stimulator morning and night.	✓ Apply morning and night.
Skin Glo	Place on clean skin and leave for 15–30 minutes. Rinse fully and place nourishing serums.	✓ Apply weekly
Reverse ageing, thicken and revitalise your skin		
Naturally A Starter	Start rebuilding and advance to stronger vitamin A as skin improves. Only advance if the skin does not feel dry.	✓ Apply 1 pump morning and night

LSM skin care products	Anti-ageing protocol How to use	When
Reverse ageing, thicken and revitalise your skin		
Naturally A Mid Strength	May commence Mid Strength after completing 2 bottles of Starter.	✔ Apply 1 pump morning and night
Naturally A Full Strength	May commence Full Strength after completing 2 bottles of Mid Strength.	✔ Apply 1 pump morning and night
Advanced Rejuvenating	Repairs skin through DNA repair and cellular stimulation. May be used with the basic trio.	✔ Apply 1 pump morning and night
Skin Growth Accelerator	Active serum designed to accelerate growth of epidermal cells. May be used with the basic trio.	✔ Apply 1 pump morning and night
Eye care		
Rejuvenating Eye Serum	May use either eye serums or both and alternate between morning and night application.	✔ Apply morning and night
Eye Nurture		
Sun protection		
Sun Defend Tinted	Nourishing anti-radiation formula to protect against the sun.	✔ Apply daily
Sun defend No Tint	Nourishing anti-radiation formula to protect against the sun.	✔ Apply daily, best 20 minutes prior to sun exposure.

To improve ageing naturally in your skin, both internally and externally, strategies are best to be adopted. Given time you will find, as I have, that your skin will defy the normal ageing process and you will feel more youthful and your skin rejuvenated.

SUMMARY

❧

I n my clinical experience, over the last 15 years I have found that any skin condition is a reflection of your internal health when there is a lack of harmony. When the body is in balance, the skin expresses vitality, health and a beautiful glow. However, the skin suffers whilst an imbalance is present.

We cannot always be aware of the impact that our regular choices and habits in food, lifestyle activity, skin care and relationships will have on our bodies. It is only in retrospect that we learn what works and what doesn't.

This book is an accumulation of all the research, clinical work and clients that I have seen over the last 15 years and the clinical outcomes that I have achieved for these clients.

Being educated within the medical model, I was always diagnosing the condition so I could fix it. However, as you will have seen in this book, there are a lot of similarities between different skin conditions and should you wish to apply the principles of good health, so too will your skin mirror that given adequate time for healing and change.

"So why use skin care; isn't diet enough?" I am often asked. Well, for me, I know that my skin is exposed to the environment and the elements on a daily basis and suffers when my body is out of balance, so I want to not only protect it but rejuvenate it! I also know that my skin is the last organ, together with the hair and nails, to get a nutrient supply, so it makes perfect sense to use topical nutrients to improve the skin's health, maintain moisture and support its resilience. This is why my skin care programme came about, together with the nutritional and investigative approach.

I hope that when you apply this information to your life, you too can enjoy health, vitality and beautifully glowing skin.

REFERENCES

1. Lee J. *Optimum Health Guidelines*, 4th edn. BLL Publishing Sebastopol, CA, USA, 1999.

2. LaValle J, Lundin Yale S. *9 Keys to Optimal Health: Cracking the Metabolic Code*. Laguna Beach, CA, USA: Basic Health Publications Inc, 2004.

3. Wartian Smith P. *What You Must Know about Women's Hormones*, 1st edn. New Hyde Park, NY, USA: Square One Publishing, 2010.

4. Samvat R, Osiecki H. *Sleep, Health & Consciousness — A Physician's Guide*. Eagle Farm, Qld, Australia: Bio Concepts Publishing, 2013;47–48.

5. Osiecki H. *The Nutrient Bible*, 8th edn, Eagle Farm, Qld, Australia: Bio Concepts Publishing, 2010.

6. Viewed 30 September 2015, https://www.floridacrystals.com/content/126/the-history-of-sugar.aspx

7. Viewed 30 September 2015, http://www.nytimes.com/2011/04/17/magazine/mag-17Sugar-t.html?_r=0

8. Viewed 30 September 2015, http://blogs.scientificamerican.com/brainwaves/is-sugar-really-toxic-sifting-through-the-evidence/

9. Viewed 30 October 2015, http://thepaleodiet.com/exactly-eating/

10. Viewed 29 September 2015, http://www.wholevegan.com/refined_sugar_history.html

11. http://www.forbes.com/2008/07/28/skin-cancer-hotspots-forbeslife-cx_avd_0728health.html

12. Viewed 15 May 2014, https://www.patrickholford.com/advice/hormone-problems-can-be-balanced-naturally

13. Viewed 20 May 2015, http://www.scientificamerican.com/article/vitamin-d-deficiency-united-states/

14. Brownstein D. *Iodine: Why You Need It, Why You Can't Live Without It*, 4th edn. West Bloomfield, MI, USA: Medical Alternative Press, 2009.

15. Viewed 20 November 2015, www.Drmercola.com/thyroid health

16. Buttermints recipe (page 163). Viewed 20 April 2014, http://www.damyhealth.com/2012/07/top-30-best-raw-desserts.

17. Raw super bliss balls recipe (page 162). Viewed 20 April 2014, https://therawfoodkitchen.com.au/raw-food-recipes

18. Roast vegetable salad recipe (page 143). Viewed 16 March 2014, http://www.bbcgoodfood.com/recipes/category/healthy

19. Chocolate brownies recipe (page 161). Viewed 16 June 2015, http://www.jamieoliver.com/recipes/category/special-diets/dairy-free

20. Pancakes recipe (page 134). Viewed 30 May 2014, http://www.bbcgoodfood.com/recipes/collection/dairy-free

21. Viewed 10 July 2015, http://elanaspantry.com/dairy-free-recipes

22. Viewed 15 June 2015, http://www.webmd.com/sleep-disorders/features/9-reasons-to-sleep-more

23. Viewed 30 September 2015, http://www.freedieting.com/tools/calorie_calculator.htm

24. Bliss ball recipe (page 162). Viewed 20 April 2015, http://www.damyhealth.com/2012/04/superfood-goddess-bites-super-balls

25. Viewed 20 June 2014, http://www.bodyandsoulcom.au/weight+loss/lose+weight/insulin+resistance+may+be+making+you+fat, 7603

26. Good fats (page 166). Viewed 20 June 2014, http://www.goodfats101.com/fats-101/omega-9s/

27. Food colourings and flavour enhancers (Table 11 page 164) Viewed 30 June 2015, http://www.betterhealth.vic.gov.au/bhcv2/bhcarticles.nsf/pages/Food_additives

28. Viewed 25 October 2015, http://www.betterhealth.vic.gov.au/bhcv2/bhcarticles.nsf/pages/Breathing_to_reduce_stress

29. Viewed 25 October 2015, http://www.ncbi.nlm.nih.gov/pmc/articles/PMC3051853/

30. Viewed 16 March 2014, http://www.intuition-physician.com/category/healthy-weight/

31. Viewed 20 February 2015, http://www.barefoothealing.com.au/v/how-could-earthing-help-me/23

32. Viewed 20 February 2015, http://articles.mercola.com/sites/articles/archive/2012/11/04/why-does-walking-barefoot-on-the-earth-make-you-feel-better.aspx

33. Ober C, Sinatra ST, Zucker M. Earthing: the most important health discovery ever, 2nd edn. 2014.

34. Wartian Smith P. Why you can't lose weight. Square One Publishing, 2011.

35. Viewed 30 November 2015, http://www.jcadonline.com/2008/09/the-role-of-diet-in-acne-and-rosacea/

36. Viewed 30 November 2014, http://thepaleodiet.com/dairy-milking-worth/#.VluLBK2hcSk,

37. Viewed 30 November 2014, http://www.leakygut.co.uk/Dysbiosis.htm,

38. Viewed 25 November 2014, http://www.culturesforhealth.com/milk-kefir-grains-composition-bacteria-yeast

39. O'Meara C. *Changing habits Changing lives, The Australian way to good food, better health and more energy.* 2007.

40. Sellman S. *Hormonal Heresy: What Women Must Know About Their Hormones.* 2001.

41. Roberts A. *The Complete Human Body Book.* London, UK: Dorling Kindersley Limited, 2010.

42. Wilson J. *Adrenal Fatigue: The 21st Century Stress Syndrome.* Smart Publications, 2002.

43. Johnson B *Transform your Skin Naturally.* Active Interest Media, Inc, 2010.

44. Fife B. *Oil Pulling Therapy, Detoxifying and Healing the Body Through Oral Cleansing.* US: Piccadilly Books, 2008.

45. Pugliese MD, Peter T. *Advanced Professional Skin Care* Medical Edition, The Topical Agent, LC. 2005.

46. Turner D. Iodine — *Thyroid & Cancer: A Question of Balance.* [Webinar]. 2013.

47. Abraham GE, Flechas JD, Hakala JC. *Orthoiodosupplementation: Iodine Sufficiency Of The Whole Human Body.* The Original Internist 2002;9:30–41.

48. Patrick L. *Iodine Deficiency and Therapeutic Considerations.* Alternative Medicine Review 2008; 13(2).

49. Wardlaw G, Hampl J, DiSilvestro R. *Perspectives on Nutrition,* 6th edn. McGraw Hill Publishing, 2004.

50. *The Prevalence and severity of iodine deficiency in Australia.* Prepared for the Australian Population Health and Development Principal Committee of the Australian Health Ministers advisory Committee, December 2007.

51. Kapil U. Health Consequences of Iodine deficiency. Sultan Qaboos University Medical Journal December 2007; 7(3):267–272.

52. Tim Spector,The Diet Myth, Orion publishing Group Ltd, 2015

53. Giulia Enders, Gut the inside story of our body's most under-rated organ, Scribe Publications, 2014

54. Robynne Chutkan MD,The Microbiome Solution, Scribe Publications, 2015

55. Thomas G Guilliams Ph.D., Supplementing Dietary Nutrients, A guide for Healthcare practitioners, Point Intsitute, USA 2014

56. Thomas G Guilliams Ph.D. with Roni Enten M.Sc., The Original Prescription How the latest scientific discoveries can help leverage the power of lifestyle medicine, Point Institute, USA 2012